Flying With One Wing

My Lifelong Journey With Chronic Illness

I0022806

Eliza Tyler

Irish Lass Publication

Dedication

To my mother, Pat, for her unconditional love, support and never-ending encouragement in some of life's most difficult situations.

To my daughter, Hillary, for being my advocate and always having my back. Thank you for laughing with me through the struggles and joys of life.

Table of Contents

Preface i

Overview of the Disease... 1

Born in a Small Town.. 3

Dynamics 5

Isn't Life Strange 10

Family Life.. 14

When We Were Young 19

Healthcare Coverage and Complications.................... 22

Marriage and Divorce Years 27

Post Divorce 30

Relationships - 1... 36

A Little Understanding 40

Post-Partum 42

Complications of Stress 43

Spiritual Guidance.. 47

Relationships – 2 49

Financial Stress 51

The Big Move 53

Going Back to School 60

Trail of Great Loss 2006 – 2008................................ 64

My Biggest Loss.. 69

Lost, Alone, and Running Out of Options 72

Stem Cell Mission... 74

Always Something... 78

Re-think – Re-evaluate 80
Taking a Leap of Faith.. 82
My First Treatment 87
From the Outside Looking In 91
Life is looking up? 108
The Hits Keep Coming.. 113
The Hit that Changed My World.................................. 115
Accident Aftermath.. 117
Hillary's Outlook on the Situation............................... 121
Healthcare and Justice.. 131
Where I Am Today 135
My Opinions and Hopes for the Future........................ 138

Preface

I STARTED THIS project several years ago after my stem cell treatments and a head-on motor vehicle accident where I suffered a closed head trauma (TBI). I will honestly admit this has been a challenge to complete with many health issues coming to the forefront since.

This is my story of living with a chronic autoimmune disease known as Type 1 Diabetes. On the following pages you will come with me on the day-to-day challenges of balancing blood sugars and living the best life possible while also coping with life's ups and downs. I will share my childhood, family dysfunction, relationship turmoil, other health issues and a few stories from friends and family. I will also share my hopes for research and development of a potential cure so that one day, perhaps, there will be no more T1D.

Overview of the Disease

I'D LIKE TO begin with an overview of what Type 1 Diabetes is and the complications that can occur as the years pass. The prognosis I was given in 1972, at the age of nine years-old was grim for a child to absorb.

Type 1 diabetes is an autoimmune disease. Autoimmune as defined by Webster's Dictionary is: as of, relating to, or caused by auto-antibodies or T-cells that attack molecules, cells, or tissues of the organism producing them.

Autoimmune diseases include a list of life altering, chronic, and potentially fatal diagnoses to include: Type 1 Diabetes, MS, rheumatoid arthritis, lupus, and a host of others. All of these diseases come with a long list of complications and hold life altering changes to one's body, mind and spirit.

In Type 1 diabetes (T1D) the immune system attacks, for still unknown reasons, the beta cells of the pancreas. These are the cells that produce insulin, which is the needed hormone to break down sugars and carbohydrates in the body to utilize energy. When the attack occurs there are as described in the chapters ahead, signs and symptoms that would indicate the disease. Symptoms can include: extreme thirst, frequent urination, weight loss, fatigue, etc., and if left untreated can lead to coma and death.

There are several subtypes of diabetes, Type 1, Type 2, and gestational (pregnancy) being the most well-known. The most common type is Type 2, or adult onset. These people make up the majority of those afflicted. Type 1 diabetics (juvenile onset) only make up 5-10% of the diabetic population. For myself, this has caused some major disagreements with people who insist I could be cured if only I applied myself and did a number of often outrageous rituals. I did not bring this on myself, I was only 9-years-old. I was not an overweight child, I did not eat excessive amounts of sugar, etc., the list goes on and on. My body/immune system attacked itself, period. There is currently no cure, only management in which we can use to maintain as normal a blood glucose level as possible. For Type 1's, myself included, the treatment is insulin via injections or pump therapy.

It was early in my diagnosis that I was described as a "Brittle Diabetic." Defined by Tabor's Medical Dictionary as follows: Diabetes mellitus that is exceptionally difficult to control. The disease is marked by alternating episodes of hyperglycemia (highs) and hypoglycemia (lows). The etiology of this diagnosis can be many. Insulin is not absorbed appropriately, or well; insulin requirements vary rapidly, exercise, diet, or medication schedules vary, or physiological or psychological stress is persistent.

There is a plethora of information that can be found on the internet through a vast number of legitimate websites.

JDRF, founded in 1970 is a good place to start. www.jdrf.org

Diabetes Research Institute out of Florida, is making progress in the clinical trials of what may one day be a potential cure using stem cell knowledge. https://diabetesresearch.org

Clinical trials are also a way of being a part of the cure. https://clinicaltrials.gov

These are my go-to sites for disease information.

With the above descriptions in mind, let's move forward through my journey of speed bumps and potholes.

I hope you enjoy the read.

Born in a Small Town

WHAT I REMEMBER from my childhood, prior to the age of nine, seemed normal to me. Small town, little neighborhoods, family-oriented cul-de-sacs, everyone knew everyone.

As a child, I remember my father was a truck driver for a grocery chain until he was diagnosed with Ankylosing Spondylitis (AS) in the early 70's. AS is also an autoimmune disease for which the spine fuses together along with systemic inflammation and a stiffening of the body. My Dad was a very negative individual. He had a drinking problem and when he stopped working due to his disease, his negativity seemed to spiral and chaos was the norm.

My mother was an amazing soul. She was always working, inside and outside the home. Despite disagreements we would have in life, she was always my mentor, my best friend and advocate. She did the best she could with what she had to work with. At times, that wasn't much.

I am one of six children between them. I fall fourth in line, and I am the only girl. My three older brothers were all born in the city of Boston where my parents lived and worked early on in their marriage. Upon my birth in Concord, MA in July 1963 we resided in the town of Maynard. Two younger brothers would come along in 1966 and 1968 respectively. BOOM, a nuclear family.

My mother put up with an immense amount of bullshit regarding my fathers drinking, the musings of my brothers, and a childhood of her own which was riddled with its own heartache and loss. My siblings, I have learned in recent years, have a whole set of their own issues from their childhood, which in my opinion, they clearly have not yet dealt with or been able to move past. Those would be their issues, their obstacles.

This is my story. My life. The encounters I will describe can be very dark. I believe this may have been where I developed what has been described as "gallows" humor. This humor has worked very well for me through the years.

I have three older brothers who range from 12 to 7 years older than myself, E, MJ, and CW.

My two younger brothers, ED and JJ, were always at each other, a constant bickering is what I recall. "Mom, he's looking at me." Always getting into trouble from the time they were toddlers. I have no doubt in my mind that once I was diagnosed that their world become somewhat chaotic as well.

There are a multitude of books written on the subject of sibling placement. They have all played a role in the person I am today, but not for the reasons for which some may think.

Dynamics

IN THE SUMMER of 1972, my best friend at the time and her family had moved away. I was really devastated. We spent so much time together, swimming at her home, playing dolls, riding our bikes, etc. Yes, there were other kids on the block, but for me, chaos and happenings that could be heard through the neighborhood kept me sort of secluded from most. I always felt somewhat cautious of people as a child. Not unusual according to my mother. She would often tell me that the only man, other than my father, that I would go near as a child was my Godfather, Pete. Anyway, that fact, did not keep me from being observant.

In September of 1972 I began the 4th grade and was only in school a couple of weeks or so when I came down with a "virus." This virus seemed to go on forever. I remember my mother taking me to the pediatrician several times over the course of a couple of weeks, as I grew weaker and weaker. I was not getting any better. In fact, I lost so much weight that I looked emaciated. We were not rich by any standards. My father had been declared disabled in 1972 and my mother was the only one working. Running to the doctor every time one of us had the sniffles was out of the question. Doctor Spock was my mother's best friend.

The family dynamics at the time, that I recall, was that E had graduated from high school the year before and had recently become engaged to his high school sweetheart. MJ was a senior in high school and was scheduled to graduate the following year. CW was a sophomore and up to his eyeballs in a new girlfriend every other month. The little ones, ED and JJ were just 5 and 6.5-years-old at the time.

After one such visit to the pediatrician, a man I was not super fond of to begin with, he's telling my mother that we just need to let the virus run its course. Home again we go. I am unaware of how much time had passed, but my last vivid recollection of this incident was a trip to the local Kmart with my mom, CW and the two youngest. I had become SO thirsty all the time. I couldn't get enough fluid in my body to quench it. I picked up a 2-litre bottle of Coke as we walked through the door and proceeded to pound it back like water. By the time we made it to the shoe department at the back of the store I had to use the bathroom. We got home and I went to bed and this went on for a few more days with me becoming weaker and weaker and excessively lethargic. My stomach hurt SO badly I reverted to the fetal position. The pain was like a knife being twisted. I kept throwing up any sort of real food, all I wanted was fluid. The last thing I remember was collapsing in the hallway to the bathroom. At that point I had begun to fade in and out of consciousness. So weak I couldn't walk without help.

Getting no real answers from the pediatrician or the local emergency room, my mother told my dad to get the car, we were going to Children's Hospital in Boston.

Boston was about 30 miles east of where we lived. Back then there were no seat belt laws and there was no EMS or town ambulance services. I was placed across the back seat of our brown Chevy station wagon, in and out of consciousness on the trip to the city. My dad did most of the driving back then, and by the time we arrived at Boston Children's Hospital I was unconscious. I had slipped into a coma.

Now, shit got really weird for me as a 9-year-old girl never having really been sick other than the common cold and the chicken pox. I'm guessing, as all my memory was now on the odd happenings I was experiencing in my unconscious state. This is where it was all so clear. I am clearly unconscious and non-responsive. Just a little girl's body laying lifeless on the gurney. Hold on now, I am clearly watching the happenings being done to my body, however, I am not moving! I am suspended on the ceiling with a heavyset black woman. YEP, I'm thinking something not right is going on here. I could very clearly hear everything that was going on. The humming of the lights, the voices of doctors telling my parents that they should prepare as I "may not make it through the night."

At that moment, I saw my father hang his head, turn and exit the room, leaving my mother standing alone and looking devasted. My father never returned to the inside of a hospital room with me again until I gave birth to my daughter in 1989! This was October 7, 1972. So here I am suspended on the ceiling with this unknown woman and we are listening to the doctor tell my mother that I am in a "diabetic coma." "She's in bad shape." My mother says, "I have five other children at home." Doctors again tell her, "She may not make it through the night."

The woman sitting with me in this celestial space, a state of unreal is asking me questions. "Are you sure you want to leave her?" "She looks like she needs you." "You need not come if your are not ready." "You have a life to do things." What the hell is that supposed to mean to a 9-year-old? Whatever I may have thought at the time, I NEVER mentioned this happening to anyone until years later for fear of being locked up in the nuthouse. Who would have believed this sort of mumbo-jumbo coming from a child? I do know that after this celestial encounter, I felt no fear, only calm and comfort. I was feeling no pain even as I watched the doctor and staff poking me with numerous needles, tubes, and other probing apparatus.

I do not know how long I remained in the coma, but I do know I spent close to a month in the hospital. I was changed forever and always felt different than I had prior to getting sick. This would become the biggest understatement ever in regard to my life and how I would live it.

After the long hospitalization and all the new ways of life, I returned home and had to attempt going back to school. ARrrggg … I had mounds of school work that needed to be completed. Not much of the school work sent home got attention while I was hospitalized, and in looking at the pile I had no desire to move forward. The changes in my life that I had to adjust to were just beginning.

Now mind you, back in 1972 there were no glucose meters, no insulin pumps, but disposable syringes were just coming to light. My days consisted of my mother waking me, or attempting, it always seemed like such an effort to get going. In hindsight, my blood sugars were likely either astronomically high or low. There seemed to be no happy medium, which would eventually gain me, in the medical community, the title of "brittle." I hate that term! I would get up and proceed to the bathroom, pee in a cup, do the whole test tube thing attempting to see where my blood sugar was at. My mom would then call the pediatrician for insulin dosing for the day. In the beginning, there was only one shot per day consisting of a regular and a long-acting insulin, but that regimen would change in the future. I would then attempt to do the school day. Years later we would learn that this method was not all that accurate in the realm of blood sugar readings.

Before my diagnosis I really loved school. I loved learning new things and letting my imagination take me to places I would most likely never get to see, and do things I may never get to do, I dreamt of going to college. After the diagnosis, that didn't always work out. I often had a hard time focusing, in large part due to my blood sugar dropping. I remember the school nurse like it was yesterday. She saw me in her office almost every day, every other day at best. I can't imagine that the diabetic kids of today have it any easier even with all the technology available in treatments, i.e., glucose meters, CGMs and insulin pumps. Again, in hindsight and with the Edmonton Protocol of the early 1980's, much has been learned. All those things I thought in my mind as a young child/teenager have proven true. Such as; dipstick testing and test tube testing were not remotely close to a real-time reading. Thus, medication was dosed on such readings, which created issues. I did the best I could to stay engaged, to learn, and to keep up with the other kids. But, yes, there is always a but! I don't know how I came across, or if I exuded the intelligence, I knew I had, but I just couldn't keep up physically, mentally, or emotionally.

I remember a few happenings upon returning back to school that would forever mold my thoughts of others. There were a few kids whom I always thought of as friends, but they stopped playing with me. Whispers of yet others stating "she's contagious." Well, that chip that started being dug out while coming to grips with this shit was really becoming a tad jagged. Kids can be so cruel, always have and always will. I learned pretty fast that I could mask some of my pain with humor. I adopted humor and I am actually pretty good at it, with a splash of sarcasm. I was not a fan of kissing ass as a kid, and I certainly do not play the ass kissing game today.

Isn't Life Strange

THE DIAGNOSIS OF juvenile diabetes, now referred to as Type 1 diabetes had changed life as I knew it and it was about to get real on discharge home.

While in the hospital I raised a little hell in the attitude and behavior department. I felt as I was being held hostage by the adults. I was being taught to inject an orange, how to eat on an exchange program, exercise, food limitations, testing of urine, and the dreaded insulin injections, of which I would put up a huge fight in the days, weeks, and months to come. Regulating me was what they were attempting to do before being discharged home. I was taking it all in, but not without some major irritation and a lot of fearful anger. Right in front of me, as if I were deaf, a doctor makes the statement to my mother, "she'll be lucky to see the age of 21, so let her be a kid." WTF – again, what is a 9-year-old supposed to make of a comment like that? It was, after all, 1972 an era for which the children were to be seen and not heard. The entire time I am growing massive resentment, I am angry, and I am pretty sure injecting this orange is a whole lot different than shoving it into my own flesh. The proverbial chip had been chiseled and I could, and would make life miserable in the future for many. I'm sure of this fact, but no one felt the brunt of my attitude and behaviors more than my mother.

After returning home, I could feel the changes. I did NOT like any of it, not one bit. I could figure out the food stuff. I remember my mother telling people, "Thank God, Binky understands this exchange program." I may have understood it, but again, I didn't like it. I felt overprotected, the focus of everyone's attention, I did not like it. Did I say I did not like it?

Life as I knew it just a month or so prior was gone. I don't really recall much of childhood prior to it now. I remember that my brothers taught me to ride a bike, played in the snow with me, went ice skating, left the neighborhood on our bikes when we were told not to, the usual kid stuff. Some family visits from aunts and uncles occurred on a weekly basis. There had been a couple of deaths prior to diagnosis that really made an impact on me. This current loss I was feeling was quite different and I had no idea how to explain it. I couldn't verbalize it and I certainly had no clue how to navigate the changes. Life became a blur and now I was forced to deal with all this crap … or die! The death line would be used as a form of threat by many in authority as time went on. At least that was how I saw it from my position in the game. "You need to do it or you will die!"

I would find myself returning to the encounter with the black woman in the ER over and over in the years to come. Now, mind you, I don't recall even knowing any people of color back then. I know a year or two later there was a black family that moved to town and I did become friends with the youngest daughter, and I fell in love with their Mom. She often exuded the image of the woman on the ceiling with me. She was fun, energetic, real and loving. I still to this day think of her and often with much wonder and gratitude. A near death experience or out of body experience is often what it is referred to today. I still felt as this encounter had changed me and at the time I couldn't state why. I can only imagine what people thought of me at this time. A snotty little brat, prone to major mood swings and a lot of attitude. I am sure of it. Although there were people who did not hesitate to tell me what they thought, there were others who I have often wondered what their perspective was of me and my behaviors, some of which were uncontrollable and I had no idea how to cope with them.

Although I had taken dance lessons since the age of 2 or 3-years-old, as I moved ahead a couple of grades, I attempted sports and a couple of lame attempts at gymnastics. That certainly placed an ugly face of reality in my way. At age 12, I played softball in a town league, not very well, but I tried. As I entered middle school (grade 6-8) I had my issues. I struggled with low self-esteem, didn't feel as though I fit in very well anywhere. I was not a fan of the "cliques" that are formed at this age and would discover that they linger on well past high school. I found myself becoming a loaner. I met a girl in the 6th grade who would become a life-long friend. We are, to this day, still friends in spite of living on different coasts and often going a few years with nothing more than our annual birthday wishes.

Also, at this time, I played field hockey for the school. I really enjoyed it, until I didn't. This sport gave me a place to express my anger and hostility. Again, I never felt very good at any of these activities with a few very vivid memories of my blood sugar dropping and wondering if I could continue to stand up, never mind run. I rarely had anything on my person to remedy these episodes of low blood sugar. These episodes if you will, would drastically influence who I would allow into my life and how deep. No doubt a practice that has played a role in my relationships over the years. I did attempt various activities, but always found my way back to dance. Dance to me was a method of expression where I could play out whatever emotion I was feeling be it dramatic, fun, whimsical, or deep and dark. I continued to dance until I was about 15 in a manner of disciplined instruction.

The whole up and down of blood sugar and the role it played on my moods and coordination was at times overwhelming. When my blood sugar was low, I would sweat profusely, shake, and often become totally disoriented. After a glass of orange juice and the trusty peanut butter on graham crackers it would come back up into normal range. At that point I would just feel like shit and want to sleep. If I couldn't sleep, I would become incredibly cranky. Not at all a nice person. As a child, there are a lot of photographs where I have this God-awful look on my face. As I got older and we would look back at some of these photos, my mom often stated, "Binky always looks like she got a whiff of something bad!" Charming, right? One photo in particular comes to mind. When my oldest brother was getting married for the second time, I don't recall the year, but we were up in Maine and having a reception brunch at a hotel when my blood sugar began to dump. FLASH … and there it is. I looked shit-faced and I wasn't even old enough to drink. Totally wiped out from the excitement of the day, the sweat pouring out of me and my outfit now soaked, and my hair out of control, I no longer felt so pretty for the festivities. This type of happening would occur over and over and over again in my lifetime, and often with the worst timing.

Family Life

FAMILY LIFE WAS already a tad chaotic when I was diagnosed. My oldest brother would tell his friends that I was going to die before I was 12-years-old, yes, a neighborhood girl told me this as an adult. In 1972-73 he was already living outside the home. MJ and CW and the two younger boys were still living at home. Dad was drinking heavily, every single night. Living in a duplex, there was an awesome family lived next door. The oldest daughter, Patty, would take me places with her, the mall, the beach and this time was something I grew to treasure. She never really seemed to treat me as others did, and to this day she holds a very special place in my heart as a sort of savior. As far as my brothers were concerned, the older boys were always good to me. No abuse, just sibling banter, etc. I felt loved and protected. He would take me to the circus, ice skating, and a few places that let's just say, Mom wouldn't have been thrilled about. When he was in high school, I would be allowed to join in on their "float parties." Float parties were a bunch of kids that would gather to socialize and make a crap-ton of Kleenex and tissue paper flowers to decorate floats for an upcoming football game or parade. I have very fond memories of some of the people who would attend these gatherings. I do feel that some of these people may have been tolerant of my presence based on false pretense, but I appreciated their kindness just the same.

The younger two brothers, well, I really didn't pay much attention as they seemed just too young and would become a major snag in the family unit with their trouble making.

I was feeling ever so smothered in the early years. Eat this, don't eat that, do this, don't do that. It would seem that my new disease status placed lots of pressures on the entire family. In the years to come, I would not help the matter as I was about to reap some major havoc and attitude of my own and it no doubt had an effect on all of those around me. Four to five years post diagnosis, I would find myself struggling on so many levels trying to find my way on this journey that no one could have prepared me for. POOF!!! I'm a teenager.

As stated earlier, I am one of six children and the only girl. My father had already been declared disabled. I knew we were no Ozzie and Harriet, but given the rest of the neighborhood, I thought it was fairly normal. I remember moving a few times as a child. Never very far, i.e., a couple of houses down, once across town. Everyone seemed to know everyone, and if they didn't, they knew someone who did. I loved my little town as a child. It was a small mill town with much diversity. We had Polish, Finnish, Irish, Portuguese, Puerto Rican and Italian neighborhoods all in this tiny town. I never thought much about what someone looked like, or how they spoke. On top of that, I met some pretty cool, amazingly smart people whom, if you listened to their stories, you could learn about other parts of the world. That was how I saw the encounters.

In the larger extended family unit, I am in all reality from another generation. I have had many cousins whom have already passed on, yet I feel that I have a valuable connection to those I remain in contact with. I am so grateful for these relationships.

As for my older brothers, they were pretty much all out of the house by 1975, with two going into the service and the oldest getting married and divorced within a year. They were good to me, but on the same hand, they all went on their own way as soon as they were old enough to do so. I am aware from conversations that have been had with them, that they had issues with my Dad, maybe my mother too. I will never know how they feel as that is their story, not mine. E, was married and out of the house. MJ would enlist in the Air Force and left home right after graduating High School. At the age of 10, it felt like abandonment, a loss I would struggle to recover from and yet, better find a way to cope. Two years later, CW would follow the same path, making the Air Force a career and returning home very infrequently over the next 25 years. He and his first wife, and their son did return from Europe in 1984 to take part in my wedding.

We had a lot of good times and there was a point in my life where I felt close to all of the older boys. That was how I perceived our relationships. When CW left, I really did feel like I was on my own now. It was 1976 when he left and I was lost. My father was still actively drinking, and very heavily. ED and JJ, well, there is an entirely different family dynamic right there. In a sense, it was if my parents had two families given the age differences, and no doubt the manner in which times changed. The two younger boys, and I never really thought about it until I was older, perhaps did suffer from a lack of attention, but ... they were always doing something that wasn't the norm, or deviant if you will. Smoking dope by age 10 or 11, skipping classes in grade school, stealing, and other things that always seemed to bring negative attention from the outside. The family unit was dysfunctional at best.

Was that my fault? Not by any means of intent, but who am I to say, I was desperately trying to find a normal for myself in a very chaotic household. It wasn't until years later when my own marriage fell apart that my mother and I opened up about things that were never said. She had regrets, and yet, it would seem my brothers never allowed her to say "I'm sorry" or "I regret ..." Some of them have held onto past hurts without ever taking responsibility for their own actions, and their methods of doing such have been at times, toxic. I refuse to take blame for someone else's understanding or lack thereof, to make them feel better, especially when they did nothing to educate themselves on what was happening to me or even attempt to understand. It seemed so much easier to run, and I do understand that to a certain level.

Denial: it was a huge resident in our home. I am sure that my mother wishes she could have denied a lot of things, if not everything, that was happening, or the added stress for which I placed on her. You see, in the beginning, upon our arrival home from BCH and learning this new life, I outright refused to take that injection! I watched my mother's hair turn whiter with gray as I added to her daily stress levels, and the nights of "sleeping with one eye and ear open."

My teenage years were tumultuous, at least for me. I hated mornings as I always felt like shit. Lethargic and cranky with the rituals at hand. I had complained about issues I noticed as my body was changing and I always got the dismissive responses as if to say, "you're just a child, what do you know"? Well, I know my body! It would turn out that all of the tools we had to test blood sugar and ketones were not even real time results. This would prove to feed some of the complications that will show up in the years ahead. Glucometers didn't come into play for me until the early 1980s.

When I was 13, I made a half-assed suicide attempt. I was told not to take aspirin, so I took a whole handful of them. That didn't work out so well. I was out with friends doing what kids did back then, and even though I felt like part of the gang, part of me was just never really fitting in. I always felt like the third wheel, feeling alone in a crowded room. I know I irritated my friends at times, probably more often than not, but they included me just the same. I could be, in the words of a dear friend's mother, a "Dr. Jekyll and Mr. Hyde" personality. Debbie and her mom, the whole family, became my family as well. Oh, the stories we would share in the years to come were amazing. I would call her mom; my daughter would go on to call her "Gramma D." She was there for me always and for everything from that point forward. She was my guardian angel here on earth in some of my darkest moments of my young adulthood.

My own mother was beside herself. She didn't know what to do with me. I was refusing to take my insulin injections. We fought about it every single morning. She would give it to me, often fighting back her own tears. Again, I wasn't making life any easier for anyone. In my early teen years, she would take me to a couple of different psychiatrists trying to find any advice on my attitude and behaviors.

When We Were Young

MY FIRST JOB was a neighborhood paper route. No big deal. Had a few low blood sugar incidents where my mom would help me complete the route. I also did the babysitting thing and enjoyed every minute of that. My second job, at the age of 14, was in a local flooring store. I really enjoyed it. Selling carpet and tile and often doing the bindings on remnants. I had a really fun relationship with the guy that hired me and to this day, we remain friendly. In 1979 I moved from the flooring store up the street to the Outdoor Store. At one point I think everyone in town worked for this store. I worked in the women's department after school and on the weekends. This is where I met my future husband even though I was not in any way, remotely attracted to him. I found him to be a childlike pain in the ass. Always sniffing me up the back stairs after punching into or out of the building, stating he liked my perfume. Up until this point, I really didn't date. I found most males my own age to be very boring and immature. Not on the same level I was. I know that sounds pretty snotty, but, it is what it is. Wayne was 4 years older than I was and at the time, I was only 15. He was very persistent and obnoxious, and my co-worker had a massive crush on him. I was not in the frame of mind where I really wanted to deal with dating anyone. There had been continued chaos on the home front with my dad's drinking, my own emotional issues, and my younger brothers causing a multitude of chaotic events often involving school and the local police. I was in a state of depression which was being blamed on hormones, unstable blood sugars and impending adulthood. I was also having issues in school. Anyway, he would tease me, sniff my perfume through the air, incessantly stating, "go out with me," "come on, go out with me." I was already aware of two other girls at the store that he was supposedly dating. I kept replying, "I'm not interested," but it didn't seem to deter him. After a few work dinner breaks ... seems we started dating, and this began what would become a 15-year roller coaster of many situations for which I had no clue how to navigate.

It was on my 15th birthday when I met his parents in a hospital room. It was our age difference that would cause some issues in our relationship, especially when I started to rebel against the wishes of my parents and older siblings.

Much of the happenings prior to our marriage I chalked up to outside influences and an immaturity factor. There were multiple deaths on his side of the family early in our relationship, one being his mother the year before we were married. Add to deaths, a couple of 30-day to 6-week long rehab stints for him: one prior and two post marriage. Again, there was a lot going on. It often seemed never ending, and much of it was stress-based drama and difficult for a teenager to navigate. I think, even now, in reflection, it was a lot! What exactly is normal?

We were together for about 6 years prior to our wedding. In that time there had been a number of blood sugar issues for which arguments or worse would ensue. He never truly understood what happened to my body during these episodes. Never seemed even remotely interested when I tried to explain. When in doubt, like the time I became unconscious on his parent's couch, he would call my mother for instructions.

We'll come back to the stress and happenings within the marriage later.

I should have graduated from High School in 1981, at the age of 17. I dropped out in March, 3 months prior to graduation. I had been missing a lot of classes, and I was just pissed off at a couple of the teachers I had. I was pissed off at the world. In any event, I had a blow up with the business teacher one day and just said, "FUCK THIS!" My mother, not being thrilled, and down right disappointed, stated I will get a job and I will get my GED, pronto! I didn't have any real issues getting a job and I took the GED in August of the same year, passed with flying colors and with topics on the exam for which I had never been taught in school. Go figure. Not the norm, but, again, what is normal?

Healthcare Coverage and Complications

AS A CHILD, it was my mother who worked outside the home as the primary bread winner. My father was on Social Security Disability and as I recall the medical insurance only covered him. My mother had worked for as long as I could remember. As a little one, she worked nights on an assembly line. As a young teenager, she was working for Digital Equipment Corporation and I know she was thankful for the health coverage with one exception: I had a pre-existing illness. That meant that before I would be covered she had to be employed with said company for one year. This tiny stipulation would play a major role in my own coverage when I became an adult at age 18. Honestly, I don't know how the woman did it. She was always on the go, and often times on very little sleep.

There were multiple hospitalizations for me over the years, at least once a year and usually around the holidays, lasting anywhere from 3 to 7 days. These stays sucked, and often involved one nurse at the local hospital for whom I would nickname "Nurse Ratchet." She would lecture me, sternly about my behaviors, diet, etc.

At age 16, I was diagnosed with **hypothyroidism.** Apparently, being told it was another autoimmune hit that goes hand and hand with Type 1. I was placed on thyroid hormone therapy. A pill. At this time, I had already started smoking cigarettes, drinking, and dabbled in the smoking of marijuana as well. When I was 17 years old I had my first major disease related complication with a retinal bleed. This scared the hell out of me! I had lost the sight in my right eye in just a blink while walking up a dark driveway. I had no clue what had just happened when everything went dark. I underwent laser coagulation surgery to stop the bleeding and cauterize the vessels. I remember not being able to lift my head for days. As if that were not bad enough, I had to be awake while they did this surgery with my head strapped in so I couldn't or wouldn't jerk my head. A couple of years later, I had to undergo the surgery again on my left eye.

As part of the disease process, I was told that new blood vessels form behind the eye and that they are not strong enough to support blood flow, so they rupture. Bloody lovely, hey?

I became very fond of my eye doctor back in Lexington, MA. He would care for my "baby blues" until I move to Arizona in 2000. When I was 17, Dr. T was fairly fresh to the whole surgical venue, but young, decent sense of humor, and not to bad to look at. For me, that was always a plus. We would develop a positive rapport and he, too, saw me through some difficult times.

My healthcare nightmares began back in 1981 when I turned 18 and became a working adult. I had a full-time job, but at the time most health insurance plans required that one year of employment to be covered due to the pre-existing illness. This began my understanding of what was to come. Over the years I would have several issues with coverage. When I was first married, in 1984, I carried my own health insurance coverage. I felt safer that way knowing what I needed to be covered. At that time, it was basically just my insulin, syringes, medications and doctor visits.

As a newly labeled adult, I had to find my own provider. That didn't go so well. The first doctor I got was a complete and total asshole! I was not about to place my life in the hands of some "Der" who was as anal retentive as this guy. Needless to say, I was most likely not the most pleasant of patients to deal with at the time. I was stubborn! A few months went by and one night I had an ER visit (there had been a few for various reasons, some brought on by my own stupidity). I was treated, reprimanded, fingers pointed, and threats of death again reiterated. My mom had been working with a woman who was also diabetic and inquired as to who she saw for care.

Enter, Melvyn. It was 1982-83 and, although we had our share of run-ins, he cared for me exceptionally well for over 18 years until I moved to Arizona. I was his challenge; I kept him on his toes. I became as fond of him, as he of I. He saw me marry, worked with me through the very difficult process of birthing my daughter, my divorce, the stressors of domestic abuse, and had tears in his eyes when we said goodbye on my move out west. I am grateful for the way he dealt with me, and especially with the humor in which I like to address these life issues. We did have a few good laughs. Laughing was a means of coping for me, and often putting others in a sense of ease which made accepting the serious with a little more relaxed approach. At other times, my humor was, and still is, looked at as my not caring about myself. Nothing could be further from the truth! My outlook is this; if I take myself SO seriously that I can't find any humor in life, that sort of approach is only going to do more damage. Let's face it, we all have the same destination, we are all going to die.

When health insurance shifted to HMOs and PPOs, Melvyn always had the diabetics back. When insurers were calling for 15-minute appointments, he was still running as much as an hour behind. To many this was a major irritation, myself included, but when someone needed the attention, and yes, at times it was me, he was there ready and willing for the challenge. His diabetic patients came first. There are not a lot, if any doctors like that today. He was open, honest, and readily available for communication and advice no matter what the issue was. I know there was more than one occasion where I pissed him off in my methods of coping with not only my disease, but those issues that came about in life, i.e., pregnancy. There were also times when I didn't have the money to pay him, he saw me anyway.

After the birth of our daughter, life started to have a bit more challenge for me. I now had this little person who was totally dependent on me being at the top of my game. Me being on the top of my game at the time meant that I gave up a lot of the partying ways we seemed to have mastered back in those days. My husband at the time, who was sober for a short period of time prior to and just post Hillary's birth, became what is known as a "dry drunk." He made my life a living hell! "You're no fun," "Why don't you party with us anymore?" HELLO!?!? There is that baby down the hall that needs someone to be responsible. Needless to say, as the next couple of years progressed, the deterioration of my marriage became evident. It didn't matter what I did, what I said, if I fought him or attempted to walk away. In his eyes, everything was my fault.

As the years have passed I have learned that just being a Type 1 has its signs of high risk happenings. It went from walking around barefoot to dental work, to surgeries, of which I have had my fair share. When I first moved to Arizona in the year 2000, the first doctor I found that would take me on as my PCP stated on our first meeting, "WOW, you have quite the record. You've had everything done but an autopsy." I sat laughing, and then recalling what an insensitive statement that was. I try to take everything with a chuckle, or at least the potential of a laugh. The fact that I can find humor in these situations, I believe, says I have a better grasp of my reality than some of these so-called medical professionals.

Since being in Arizona over the course of 23 years now, I have undergone surgeries to include; a partial hysterectomy, multiple cardiac ablations (to correct irregular heart rhythms) which intensified after the hysterectomy due to an issue with anesthesia and an underlying electrical short-circuit in my heart. I had my nose fixed due to fracture, deviated septum, and polyps in my sinuses. I had a hernia operation that turned out to be totally unnecessary. The surgeon stated afterward, "I don't think that is your problem as it was very small and really didn't need surgical intervention." My PCP at the time, a PA, who referred me for the surgery, also nearly did me in by trying to prescribe a Type 2 drug to lower my A1c. I protested and stated I would not take it, she called me noncompliant! Can you say lawsuit? Which I could have, and perhaps should have, filed in the case of doctor/medical professionals in this state alone. After one of my cardiac ablations, I landed back in the ER after only two days of being discharged only to have a doctor say, "We need to do a cardiac catheterization." "Your labs are showing damage to the heart." Well, no shit Sherlock, you just did that with the ablation. As I lay on the table who am I to fight with them? I am, as would anyone functioning alone, at the mercy of those in charge. They've got you! Once you're checked in, and they have you under their control, you pretty much have to oblige or risk not being covered for the charges of the services rendered. This has happened to me on more occasions than I care to count. I recall an ER visit in which I was taken by co-workers following what appeared to be signs of a heart attack. I landed with a doctor, who I would have future run-ins with, and disagreements with regard to my care. He ran the multitude of tests which would indicate a heart attack, and after many hours (no hospital run goes without hours of testing and waiting) on the table, he returned to tell me that everything came back normal, BUT (always one of those), "we are going to admit you because you are a high-risk patient." Well, I put up a stink telling him that if all the tests came back negative and nothing was found that I would be going home. He proceeded to tell me that this decision on my part was dangerous as I could go home and have a major heart attack and die! I told him without skipping a beat, that I could leave the hospital and get run over by one of their golf carts … and DIE!

As my story goes ahead you will hear me mention run-ins with the insurance industry and my ever changing awareness of how they really do NOT have our best interests or good health at heart.

At the tail end of my teenage years, and always with that big gray cloud over my head screaming, "You won't make 21!" I didn't always make the best decisions in my life and tossing out what I had hoped and dreamt, for a mundane existence.

Marriage and Divorce Years

IN 1984, IN spite of a whole lot of red flags, Wayne and I married. At the time, I believed we had a beautiful wedding. We had already conquered so many tough situations and made promises to each other and I discovered shortly after the union, those promises had already been broken. There were addiction issues for him that involved both drugs and alcohol, as well as his repeated cheating. In reality, I had left an alcoholic home with my father, and moved into one with Wayne. The marriage was not good from the start. Most of my happy memories come from time spent with his family. Often at gatherings, i.e., weddings, birthday parties, holiday festivities, even funerals, where he would decide he didn't want to be, so I went alone. Our relationship was turbulent to say the least. I tired, I really did, but several months into our marriage he broke my nose out of the blue for hanging the fucking toilet paper in the wrong direction! Ok, now, I was from a large family as was he. I am of the thought; you should be lucky there is paper on the roll. Our entire relationship was full of toxic behaviors that were usually fueled by alcohol and/or drugs.

In our first 5 years of marriage, I would have multiple miscarriages and often would arrive at work with bruising for which I had to cover or make up some lame excuse for "my" clumsiness. Yes, in hindsight, I was a victim of domestic abuse, both physical and emotional.

At this time, we both had jobs and often struggled with transportation as Wayne had lost his license on a couple of occasions. Getting to work became a source of irritation. As long as he was on time, and he got picked up as soon as he got out of work, my jobs didn't seem to matter. He didn't mind taking my paychecks, which I wasn't thrilled about in the first place. Again, another topic for which the 1950s mentality of "the man rules the roost" wasn't going to fly with me.

He did two rehab stints where he was out-of-state for weeks at a facility in Pennsylvania, paid for by his employer. I will admit, on these family week inclusions, I learned a LOT of how to cope and deal with addiction in life. Now, don't get me wrong, I par took in a lot of our partying in the beginning but I like to think I was growing up once we married and contemplated children.

In 1987, I became pregnant. I had traveled to Arizona with my folks as they were moving west and so that we could take a break and figure out what we wanted to do. Upon my return home to Massachusetts, at 18 weeks pregnant, we got into an argument which ended with me on the floor and him kicking me. At this point, I was very upset and with no phone couldn't call the doctor to check in. I went to his brother's house to use the phone. Well, I ended up in the ER and a D&C was performed. It was a nightmare! His degrading demeaner of telling me to be quiet in post-op, there were sick people in here prompted one of my nurses to read him the riot act about this trauma and made him go to the waiting room. The baby was a boy.

Five years in, he was clean and sober for several months when Hillary was conceived. It would come to light late in the pregnancy that his extra-curricular activities were adding stress to the already stressful relationship. He was constantly barking at me that "you laugh too much." "You never take anything seriously." Those words were the furthest from the truth. As it was his behaviors, his actions, and his words that lacked any kind of love and had a deep effect on me as well as our daughter. These behaviors will and did continue until well after we divorced in 1993.

Hillary was 3 years-old when I filed for divorce. I had given him ample warnings about shit I was no longer going to tolerate. Physical violence, loud ranting ramblings about what a horrible wife and mother I was, his "girlfriend" being in our bedroom when I got home from work or school. He was always up in my face.

It wasn't long after our divorce that friends who had long passed on socializing with us as a couple, or stepped away from a relationship with me, came to the forefront again. Along with that rebirth of friendships, to this day for many, came a lot of "we knew." That hurt as well, but I get it. As a husband and wife, who would want to intrude into the personal goings on of a couple? Again, many of them were witness to or had been a target of, what I often tried to brush aside, or make light or, as "he had too much to drink", "he has to work", "maybe he forgot." It was SO much more than that. Regardless of how some of his family members may feel about me, I did the best I could with the situation and I was not about to be taken out by a selfish individual who never felt a sense of remorse or personal fault for any of his behaviors. It was not in my, nor Hillary's best interest to engage any further. I had the support I needed from certain family members on his side, to keep the family unit in some sort of union. It was not ever my intention to take Hillary or keep her from his family. That worked out for those of us focused on the big picture. To this day, I am grateful for these relationships, for I would not want to forget those good times or short-change Hillary having an extended family who does love her, even though her father did not seem to know how.

Post Divorce

IN OCTOBER 1993, my divorce became final, but the harassment, stalking, and continued verbal and emotional abuse and threats continued. Along with this came an entirely new list of issues. I was working at a local pub, the credit union, and an occasional day/evening at a salon. He was following me home from work to the point I had police escorts home from the bar at night. Lucky for me I knew many of the local officers and they grew rather protective of not only myself, but Hillary as well. There were a couple of occasions where he was even able to get into our apartment building without ringing the buzzer. I never could understand this behavior as he had long ago taken up with the "other woman." It was nerve wracking at best, and that is stating it lightly.

In the 10 years we were married there was always tension. It turned out even before we married, that he had a drinking problem. After we said, "I do" ... I almost immediately thought I had made a mistake in thinking it would change. He had promised me he would be sober the night we wed, but that became obvious to pretty much everyone except me that he was not. Again, I went from one bad household situation into another one that would bring repeated heartbreak, emotional, and often physical pain. It came to my attention that he repeatedly continued to cheat on me. I was expected to forgive and forget, as in his words, "it didn't mean anything." Sorry, but that line got old really fast, and it did nothing for my heart or my level of trust. There are several who would argue this fact, but far too many others who witnessed and kept quiet until after the divorce. There were others, still, who took active roles in deceptive behaviors while trying to play both sides of the relationship. There was physical abuse, verbal abuse, and constant beating down of my self-esteem to boost his own ego, all while blaming me for anything and everything that could go wrong in life. After the birth of Hillary, I told him, "You ever hit me in front of that child and I am done!" Well … not only did I catch him in our bed with this douche bag he made his second wife, but he hit me in front of Hillary while arguing about the said douche bag! This encounter, to my shock and dismay, was and is still remembered by our child who is now a grown adult.

Several months went by and no child support was being paid. With that came death threats. If I took him to court, he would kill me. Those were his words and they slid off his tongue on many occasions. I called his bluff and took him to court on several instances. He always had an excuse, never his fault. After a while the judge wasn't buying this behavior either. We almost always appeared before the same judge.

There was a lot of fighting. I will not say I was not at fault, as I often fought back by pushing his buttons in my defense. I then learned, through the many rehab family therapies, that I was reacting to his acting out. His reactions would not get any better when I applied some of the tools which are taught in the program, i.e., AA, NA, and Al-anon.

I attempted to move forward with a new and more positive life, still not void of the stress.

This stress, for which I had learned to internalize for Hillary's sake and my own sanity, would place new stressors on me. I had never lived on my own before this, and now I had a little person who required me to have my shit together. I started feeling tired ALL the time, and when I ate, OMG, I would feel full very quickly leading me to not want to eat at all. My blood sugars were all over the charts, from lows at 25 to highs in upwards of 400. Nothing I did seemed to make any difference. This began a long period of many doctor visits.

As referenced earlier, Type 1 comes with a long list of possible complications, many of which come on naturally with long-term disease. Add chronic stress levels and you have the perfect storm. These repeated visits to the doctor would result in many tests, some invasive and uncomfortable. I was referred to a gastroenterologist for more exams. I underwent labs, nasogastric tubing, which involved feeding a tube up my nose, down my throat, and into my stomach, and some other exams which at the time had me thinking of another book to write, "101 Ways to be Creative with Crap!" The year was 1995. When all was said and done, they came back with a diagnosis of gastroparesis. Gastroparesis is a complication of the digestive tract where the muscles that propel food through the body have become paralyzed and don't work appropriately. This causes up and down blood sugars that were now going to cause some dangerous complications. So, here come the pharmaceuticals. First was a long ride on tetracycline and some other drug to rid my gut of a bacterium known as H-pylori. I was then placed on a drug named Propulsid, a drug to promote gut motility, and I was told to buy a good blender. Encouraging, right? The Propulsid worked really well in the motility area. After being on Propulsid for 2 or 3 years, I was taken off of it abruptly as it was being pulled from the market due to cases of causing sudden death. This on again/off again roller coaster would be the norm for many years to come. After the Propulsid I was tried on Reglan, which didn't like me at all, so it was placed on the allergy list. The Propulsid being yanked off the market at this time would lead me to much research, and my not so much of a fondness for our FDA (Food and Drug Administration).

In a nutshell, I suffered from massive bouts of constipation, diarrhea, bloating, severe pain, constant heart burn, and acne! Acne!! I had such great skin as a teenager and here I was 32-years-old and I have zits! I was a toxic nightmare, going as long as two weeks without taking a dump (bowel movement).

About this time, 1996 or so, I had an episode while driving where my heart started racing out of control. I was really scared. Now mind you I was with a sister-in-law at the time, driving back from Boston when the road started to become very fuzzy. I felt disoriented, hot, and visually out of whack. One would think that she would have taken over the driving when I said I wasn't feeling right and had just shot across two or three lanes of traffic. She dropped me off at my apartment and I called my mom. My mother met me in the ER where I was told it was a cardiac arrhythmia. Great, just what I needed, something else on the plate that was already overflowing. This led to a workup and a comment that "it's common in women your age, nothing to worry about." I didn't find that to be overly comforting at the time given I was only 33-years-old. Needless to say, after that ride, niece and nephews from that branch of the family were not ever in my driving bubble again. That shows some serious faith, doesn't it? My PCP started me on a couple of ACE inhibitors to try and regulate the rhythm and keep my heart from doing that bizarre dance anymore. These drugs were horrible in the side effect department, and I eventually stopped them. The erratic beating of my heart would continue off and on until 2005-2006.

The mid to late 90s for me would hold a lot of ill time. I was always fatigued, exhausted, and not sleeping well with high pain levels, not eating well, and still trying to work so I at least had some money coming in. Yes, that money thing or lack thereof can really cause some stressful situations. My loving ex-husband and all his threats were causing major problems for me in caring for Hillary. It came to the point where something had to be done. I hired an attorney with the help of in-laws and took him to court. Mind you, he had been threatening me since the divorce court appearance, that if I ever took him to court or made an issue about child support, he would kill me. I believed this as he was not a nice person when things didn't go his way. However, a child, his child, was suffering and I was getting tired of covering his ass and his lame excuses for not making that $75/week payment. Yes, $75 dollars was all he was ordered to pay based solely on his telling the court he didn't have a job, even though he seemed to have the funds to purchase a diner!

Another court appearance, several arrests, a couple of episodes where the state drained his bank accounts, and he placed his diner in the "other woman's" name, which left us out in the cold again. This vicious cycle would go on for years, even after our move to Arizona, with back child support never being paid.

The late 90s started to bring about change; some good, some not so promising. In 1997, I met a wonderful man. He would be the first man who would show me that I was not only lovable, but fun to be with. I totally enjoyed our time together, which included a month-long stay in Europe at the end of our relationship. He was SO incredibly good to both me and Hillary, loving and so respectful. To this day Hillary will bring up times we spent together in which it was all love and laughter. It was a 2 year time period in which both Hillary and I had a restored faith in man. It was a difficult end because it was such a wonderful relationship. It had to end for a couple of reasons, one being trans-Atlantic relationships with an ex that is hell bent on creating problems. This was not something I wanted any of us to be involved in. We parted ways on a healthy and adult note. I believe it was a first for me, and it taught Hillary that good people will come and go in our lifetimes, and they should be cherished for the lessons we learn.

About this time, 1998, I was told that I should put my affairs in order. I wish I could say I was devastated, but I had been expecting this announcement years prior. I had dodged that proverbial bullet. I began to do a lot of reading and research into options I may have to turn the situation around. I came across the insulin pump. I had been asked while pregnant in 1988/89 at the Joslin Clinic in Boston if I wanted to take part in a trial they were doing with the pump in pregnant women. When I saw the size of this thing, I opted out. At this time though, 10 years later, it was looking as it was really the only thing out there I had to try with the potential to stabilize me. So, I approached the doctor with it. His first response was a hard "No!" He felt I was not disciplined enough to do the required glucose testing involved in wearing a pump, which involved testing (pricking), my finger 6-8 times per day. I will admit, he had a point, and I was scared to death. His second reason, he had no other patients on a pump, therefore, having no idea what was involved. In my usual, pushy manner I researched, called the company, got the people and info needed, and approached him again. We went forward with placing me on a pump in February of 1998. At this time, I was in above mentioned relationship with Joe. He did not have a clue about my diabetes, only that I had been having some health issues. Being placed on the pump involved me coming off the long lasting insulin which had been part of my regimen since the beginning. That was pretty scary being as I lived with an 8-year-old. It was a 3 day process of weaning me off the insulin usage I was accustomed to and then being placed on the pump that uses a short acting insulin on a constant basal drip.

The pump was a Godsend. A piece of modern technology that gave me a sense of freedom on so many levels. It was priceless! Life was still a hell ride in many aspects, but blood sugars began to stabilize a bit with far less highs and drastic lows. The relationship I was in became that much closer when he refused to allow me to blow him off, and eventually told me that he completely understood as his mother was a diabetic.

Up until this time I had been on multiple injections a day with a combination of insulin, short and long acting.

Relationships - 1

RELATIONSHIPS, OF ALL kinds, require us as humans to give and take. From my own perspective, to have a relationship with me on a deep level is a challenge at best. Relationships are not just a man and a woman, or a couple, but of all the relationships we encounter in our life time.

Dating for me was awful! I didn't really date at all in school, I was more of a loaner. Meeting Wayne, well, I guess that was the extent of my dating as a teenager, young woman. After my divorce, I tried. Dating to me was like a really bad job interview, not a personal encounter. I really wasn't in the market for a committed relationship at this point. More than that, I didn't want anyone to know or get close to Hillary for fear of any more pain and rejection, for both of us. Not only for those reasons, I had an ex-husband that was like a bad penny. It was okay for him to go ahead, move in with the douche bag, eventually marry her, but continue to hound and harass me. My trust in people was far from healthy and I was in no place to risk any sort of unstable surroundings. Don't get me wrong, I like men! I have a couple of wonderful long time male friends with whom we can talk about anything, and a few more that now reside on "the other side." Sadly, not one has captured my heart, or been able to handle the ride or to cope with the things I have to do in my day-to-day life to simply remain part of the human race.

Type 1 is something I live with; it in no way defines who I am. That is my outlook, it more often than not is not an outlook others see

36

or can remotely place themselves in. Most just don't understand what is involved and don't care, or are afraid to learn. I find it amusing at times that people can't look past the disease and see the person who resides within me.

With that being said, I had a lot of baggage. For me, I needed to work through the unpacking that emotional baggage for myself before I could be of any love interest to someone else. Needless to say, 25+ years later, this feeling of understanding and a person of romantic, intimate love has eluded me. I often find myself laughing at this truth believing it is "their loss," but at the same time, especially as I age, it would be nice to have a partner to share life with. I hold a much higher standard today in who I will allow into my world on that intimate level. Although, many tell me I have to leave the house to meet someone nice, I have become very comfortable in my solitude. Maybe that is not a healthy outlook for some, but for myself I will no longer allow others to compromise my own well-being.

Relationships in general, have always had a sort of understanding to be had. I didn't learn this of myself until long after my marriage ended. I took vows that I held very seriously and when those vows were broken and betrayed, I lost my faith. I lost my faith in man, lost my faith in humanity, and lost my faith in the Catholic Church, and those people who took part in what I will always refer to as evil in my mind and spirit. Oh, I can forgive, but I will never forget the roles those individuals played. Now, I am no angel by any stretch of the imagination, but NEVER have I gone out of my way to hurt someone as those individuals did to me to advance their own agenda or assist a misguided soul. Yes, I have said things that I regret in the heat of any given moment. I have also spoken truths that were just too raw for some, and my approach in doing so was frowned upon. I did this a lot during and within my marriage. We had no idea how to argue or even communicate, both of us having come from a form of dysfunctional family dynamics. After the two rehab stints the spouse had to do while we were married, I clearly learned more than he did in regard to the beast of addiction, and I learned how to apply those tools in any given situation. He didn't particularly care for those applications. Even after 3 stays for addiction and alcohol related issues, I don't believe he ever used what was learned for anything more than to continue his manipulation of those he felt were "in the dark." It was his own father, whom I loved dearly, who during one of these mandatory stays (go or lose your job), gave me the airfare to attend family week at the facility in Pennsylvania, and stated to me with a serious tone of voice, "If I were you, I'd walk away now." Again, I had taken those vows seriously and I was being tested beyond belief in how far I would go before I would break them and just walk away. I was no longer a big fan of the man I married. I always thought I loved him. In the end, I didn't like him at all and it was blatantly clear he never loved me. If he did, he had a very warped method of expressing it.

Love is blind ... and so was I.

The best part of the entire relationship was the birth of our daughter, conceived during a brief period of sobriety on his part, and decent blood sugar control on mine. His method of celebrating while I was hospitalized after the C-section birth in 1989 was less than morally acceptable on anyone's radar. A phrase comes to mind, no pain, no gain. The pain and heartache grew deeper when the latest "other woman" began calling the house like this behavior was all acceptable. Again, who does shit like this?

Shortly after we were discharged from the hospital it all became very clear to me that the marriage was not going to survive. No, it wasn't the hormone rage, it was discovered that he had lost his job. When a large bill for the five-day stay for delivery and baby arrived showing NO insurance coverage! He had confessed to multiple infidelities, again, with the arrogant attitude of doing no wrong and stating "it didn't mean anything", and if I had only fulfilled my "wifely duties" it might not happen. I had heard this line of crap before. What amazed me, yes, I amazed myself, was I always thought if he, himself, had admitted his wrong doing that I would go ape shit in anger. That was not the case, as I recall quite vividly the evening he came home annihilated on God knows what and he fell to his knees in tears on the kitchen floor, like a 3-year-old, and confessed too many infidelities including the most recent indiscretion. I could not help but begin to chuckle. It was a pathetic scene and knowing I had heard this many times before with a long list of lies attached. I wasn't buying it this time. The trust had been severely damaged. It would continue for another 3 ½ years with several separations and half-hearted attempts to reconcile. It was over, and it was beyond repair, and would never work out when he began bringing home this so-called coworker who became known in my small circle as the DB. I had put up with a lot of his shit by this point and it was not going to happen in my home, in front of me or my daughter. Having his newfound girlfriend coming out of our bedroom upon my arrival home from school at night wasn't going to fly. What kind of woman does shit like this? A question I continue to ask myself at times. Respect starts with oneself. He wanted control; I was not having anymore of that. In the end, it would seem they were made for each other. He wanted to be controlling and she needed or didn't mind being controlled. No real respect for anyone, including themselves. It hurt beyond belief for several reasons, but I couldn't go on like this and I was not going to be his doormat or punching bag any longer.

A Little Understanding

I DON'T BELIEVE he ever really understood my disease, or what it entailed. Hell, he couldn't even understand his own (addiction). Again, always blaming someone or something else for him using or his excessive drinking, or any negative situation. Seems at every incident an issue with my health arose, he would call my mother and maybe an ambulance, and then disappear. When Hillary was small, he would throw temper tantrums about how I handled my insulin injections. He didn't want to see any of my supplies laying around. I outright disagreed. It was part of my life, and, as such, it was not going to be kept a secret from my children or in my home.

Hillary was almost 4-years-old when our divorce became final. Weekend trips to visit her father turned ugly fast. She was never happy. Either he blew her off altogether (not calling, not showing up), or he would pick her up, often late, and spend the rest of the weekend, their visitation time, drunk and passed out. This was Hillary's explanation to me years later when recalling her visits in therapy sessions. This was the sort of turmoil I had to deal with on a daily basis, all the while trying to reassure Hillary that she was loved, that none of this was her fault and would be taken care of, while trying hard to take care of myself. It became exhausting and overwhelming on an emotional level that eventually boiled over to affect my health. For those reasons, I was, and will be, forever grateful for the extended family members who were not opposed to me visiting and keeping the friendships we had developed alive and peaceful. Namely, his brother and his wife, and his sister and her husband, both Godparents to Hillary. What is most impressive is that none of us ever discussed him. These individuals always were there with open arms and a loving open door where all the kids just played as kids should. There were the occasional situations where the ex would show up at these homes and cause a scene and attempt to take Hillary while under the influence of something. Hillary has vivid recollections of a few of these incidents where I was not present, and those who protected her from what she feared most. Even after we moved away, these relationships remained intact despite physical distance.

Childbirth was not easy on my body. It was a ride I don't believe I could have done again with as positive an outcome as I had with Hillary. In spite of all the doctor appointments, and trips to Boston for labs, tests, restrictions placed, it was a LONG nine months. I don't think I would have survived a second time, and was more than happy being blessed with this beautiful, healthy baby girl following several miscarriages. For the entire pregnancy I had to drive to the city as the local doctors and hospital had me labeled high risk, so it was into Brigham and Women's Hospital for the duration.

Post-Partum

WITHIN A COUPLE of weeks of delivery, I began to have a lot of blood sugar fluctuations. Something no one had warned me about in the diabetic world. The fluctuating hormones caused a number of drastically low blood sugars that came on rapidly and had sent me into seizures on a couple of occasions. One afternoon, I recall not being able to talk, or move my limbs and I had lost control of my bladder. It was like I was having a stroke and I was scared to death sitting on the living room floor. When the EMTs arrived, I don't remember what was being said, but I was able to flip the bird (middle finger salute) at someone, and my mother, being behind me at this point said, "she's back". This sort of episode would happen 3 or 4 times over the next two weeks. One night while the hubby was out at a meeting, I remember watching Dynasty, and while feeding the baby it was like one minute I was there, and the next minute I was unconscious. Needless to say upon his arrival home he found me on the floor on top of the baby. I have no idea how long we had been in that state, but I took a heap of reprimand by him and on my comeback in the ER. At one point in the ER I got the same doctor twice. On my repeat visit he began yelling at me in a degrading tone. "You know every time you do this you are killing off brain cells?" Like I was doing this on purpose and that was my goal. I have encountered some real assholes in the medical field. Like just because they had the "Dr." before their name makes them some sort of authority on any given subject. Today, it is my opinion there are very few of them who even know the entire function of the body beyond their self-proclaimed specialty.

Complications of Stress

THIS PERIOD IN my life was exhausting. There was SO much added and unnecessary stress in life I was unsure of how to cope with it all. I did my best to make it all look nice to the outside world, an act I had mastered up to this point, or so I thought. I would eventually discover that most people knew of my ex's indiscretions, his personality, and his behaviors. So I guess it was I who looked like the fool always attempting to make an excuse. I have documented many of these episodes in journals over the years as a method of coping. Perhaps one day I will turn them into a tell all screenplay. If it could happen, it did happen, and usually it was I who got blamed for it. Prior to leaving the union with Hillary and very few belongings in tow, I sat for weeks on end in sweatpants staring out the sliding glass door wondering, pondering, and praying ... what do I do? Where will I go? How will I survive? It was all a new outlook, a really frightening leap into the unknown. I did it, and he helped push me to make the decision. As if life were not difficult enough for all of us, the added stresses of my crumbling marriage and wanting my child to be in a safe and loving environment was really taking a toll on my body and my mind.

In 1994 I was always fatigued. No amount of sleep made a difference; my body felt as if it were breaking down. My muscles gave out, and there was even a period where I could barely walk to the mailbox and back without being in excruciating pain. I would vomit my body hurt so bad which led to numerous trips and calls to the doctor. Melvyn was not only my endocrinologist, he was my primary care physician, and he began ordering tests and sending me off to specialists. Two years of this led to a multiple diagnosis of gastroparesis and fibromyalgia. Nothing treatment wise was really available except pharmaceuticals. The result of not being able to digest food / nutrients was creating an absolute impossible grasp on my blood sugars. It didn't seem to matter what I did, or didn't do, I was up and down like a yo-yo. On top of the physical pain, I was emotionally overwhelmed and completely drained. I became very depressed at my life status and how I would move forward. It was at this time when the evil conduct of a few led to a 72-hour hold in a psyche ward and Hillary being taken by her father. This was a devastating bottom line for me and I was forced to enter therapy. Now, anyone who truly knows me, knows that when I am pushed, I push back. HARD!

I was furious! Livid beyond belief! I was literally forced to enter therapy. I was not happy about this given the circumstances, but I now had no choice but to play by others' rules, and without my daughter. While I did undergo this task, and I still have the letter written by the therapist to enforce the inner strength I didn't realize I had. I survived and got my daughter back when the evil individuals were called out and exposed for what was trying to be done under the guise of what was best. My entire relationship with my ex was based on nothing more than how he could get back at me. I firmly believe that. Major manipulation, and he would continue to blame me for every bad thing that did not go right in his life. Taking Hillary was just another way of sticking it to me for him and his co-conspirators.

Hillary would suffer physical and emotional distress during this time period as well, distress that would follow her into adulthood. Did these individuals have any idea what they were doing? Was this all just a game to them? Who behaves in this manner? My life was not a soap opera, and I was not the cause of their misfortune. Messing with people in such a manner that can cause long-term emotional turmoil, especially to a child, is my idea of evil, or mental illness. You can draw your own conclusions. Very few people know how this effected Hillary. She was a child, and as a child, it was my job to take care of her, protect her, and make sure she had a childhood free of abuse, be it physical or emotional. You want to mess with me, have at it, but you will not mess with my child! I don't care who you are. I am forever indebted to those individuals who dedicated themselves to Hillary's happiness and well-being.

The 1990s sucked, and towards the end of the decade I was eventually declared disabled and began to collect a steady income even if small by a working comparison. With that declaration, I also had medical coverage for which would really ease some of the excessive stressors. Let's face it, being a diabetic, or having any other chronic illness can be a pricey endeavor. Hillary was now in school, which came with a couple of tough years in that she was always afraid if I dropped her at school, I, too, would not return to pick her up. Abandonment issues were what we were told she was suffering with. I assured her at every opportunity, "Momma will never leave you baby." It could be heart wrenching at times and all I could do is love her and do the best I could to make sure she felt that love and felt secure with those around her, or whose care I left her in. I never left her with strangers. She was always with my parents, or family. She spent endless hours with her cousins; her Dad's brother and his wife were like another set of parents. She would also spend time with my brothers and their families. It kept the semblance of a family unit intact. When we were all together as friends, the ex was not a topic. Again. Grateful for those interactions. Life went on doing the best we could with what we had and the gracious contributions of many others.

As the years began to pass I became more comfortable with the person I truly was, which really wasn't far off from where I started. I really don't give a shit what anyone thinks of me. When you can walk even a short distance in my shoes, then you can throw an opinion out there. I have had so many people make statements about not being able to see me putting up with the circumstances, or happenings of those 10-15 years. I have looked back on this period and wondered how myself. How did I survive? Why did I subject myself to that sort of treatment by another individual?

Through the grace of God.

Spiritual Guidance

I WAS RAISED Catholic. My mother often said to me she sort of "slacked off with the last three." So, I wasn't exposed to the church like my older brothers were. I often thought, after the encounter with the spiritual woman in the ER on diagnosis, that I must have some direct dial line to God. I do not consider myself a religious person. I gave up on organized religion a long time ago. With that being said, I do consider myself to be a very spiritual being. After that first near death experience which left me feeling a little odd in comparison to others. I had an almost inside look as to what may transpire when I leave this earth, therefore, not being afraid to die. In fact, there have been times when I wished and hoped for nothing more, with the exception of not wanting to leave Hillary behind in pain. As she has grown into an adult, become a medical professional herself, and the many discussions of said topic with my mother, she too, understands completely where I am coming from when I make statements about how I want to go, how I want to crossover, and my hopes for what she will believe when this happens. I do believe in God. I do believe that at some point I will be allowed to enter that place of peace, a place where I will be pain free, maybe even wrinkle free, and to see all those loved ones who have gone before me, and ... wait for it, all those super talented artists I never got to see here in the earthly life having the party of the afterlife!

I do not follow any organized religion. Not since going to the church for advice relating to my marriage and being told, "you said, for better or worse." Sorry, not the right answer! I have read about many religions, and pull what I need for myself, and let go of the rest. In my opinion, they are all a form of a cult in where each branch puts their own twist on the same book. I have taken directive from the Buddhism philosophy. As people, I do not feel that we need to have so many material possessions which in my mind only exudes greed. Not that I would deny anyone those joys, but I have learned, and apply it to my own life, that it does not matter how much you have, it can all be taken away in the blink of an eye. I have learned how to get by and survive with very little material possessions, and it's all good. I feel I do a pretty good job in sharing my encouragement, excitement, and enthusiasm for all those in my life who are successful in many areas of life and celebrating that joy with them. However, those material successes in no way mean I need to have it in my life. Just like getting all dressed up, my mantra is, less is best.

My advice is do what you need to do for you. Find a means of coping and being at ease with what life has given you. You need not prove anything, to anyone. I respect whatever you want to practice, and I am always willing to listen and learn. Just don't push your belief down my throat, because in all reality, you have no clue what I deal with on a daily basis, 24/7, 365 days a year.

Relationships – 2

THE CONTINUED BULLSHIT that came with the union of the ex and his new found douche-bag went on for several years. I swear he went out of his way to inflict any turmoil he could. It seems as though leaving me and our daughter to indulge with other women was not enough. No matter what the happening of the day was, it was my fault, at least that was his take. I would learn through AlAnon and family groups in his rehab stays that this was NOT my issue, it was his. The entire relationship was wrong and I was partly to blame for some of it as I could throw some hurtful and instigating digs in as well. I was young, inexperienced, and completely naïve to believe that he would change his behaviors once a commitment before God had been made. I would be told after our divorce of actions/moves he made on friends of mine, and what actually transpired the night we wed, and broken promises before it even began. In the early days, I, too, went along with the partying mentality. In the back of my mind, I only had a few years to cope. That line spoken by the doctors as a child was always a cloud in the back of my mind until I had Hillary. Then it became a fight or flight response. Once Hillary was born, in his eyes, I became boring, no longer wanting to act as if I had no one else depending on me. My feelings never did seem to matter to him, and with that, I had the push I needed to move out and take Hillary with me. That didn't go over so well and I got a good fist, slap, and push to show me who was in control. Fuck, even the guy that was the maintenance man at the apartment complex where we were living at the time voiced a concern for Hillary's and my well-being and safety. With the help of my youngest brother, JJ, I moved out and filed for divorce. There was no talking to him, as always, discussions were one-way: his way. I'm sorry, he was a bully!

Financial Stress

I HAD THREE jobs at this point in the mid-90s, just trying to keep a roof over our head as he outright refused to pay child support. A whopping $75/week and didn't want to pay it. He went out of his way to make it look like he didn't have any income. Funny, a person with no income can buy a dining establishment. After I got the state involved and his bank account got drained a couple of times, he got tossed in jail, and he placed everything in the douche bag's name. When he died, he was over $30k in debt to us for back child support. Add to that all the emotional abuse he inflicted on both Hillary and myself, and yet, some still hold me to blame. I am aware of at least three individuals that would, and do, continue to blame me … for what, is what I would really like to understand. You can only help someone who wants to be helped, and he was NOT one of those people.

Those who felt I kept Hillary from her father have no idea what went on. NONE! Those who enabled his behaviors are as guilty as he was. It went on and effects of such continue to linger today. It was brought to our attention that a company for which he had worked prior to and during our early marriage was in a legal matter for toxic waste and paying families for which someone became or died from any number of illnesses and cancers. Well, according to the FEDS, the CDC, and some other agency, Hillary, as his only biological child, was not entitled to the claim, but the douche bag was! She didn't even know him back then. According to an attorney out of Boston who consulted with Hillary, said it was a messed-up law dating back decades. Her father's behaviors and actions in such matters were not secret to the powers that be, yet, they always seemed to get away with not doing what's right.

Now, I could very well blame my encounters with cancer on this job of his, or his actions at said job. But, the fact of the matter is this, he was behind on child support, he inflicted undue emotional abuse on his daughter from the time she was a toddler and SHE was the rightful person whom should have received the payout. The entire situation, from start to finish, is and was beyond disgusting. I should feel bad for people like this? I don't think so and Karma can't catch their asses fast enough for me. In a sense, Karma has already proven that what goes around, comes around. I'm happy to state that I have even been witness to some of these karmic, cosmic happenings.

In a nutshell, I still had more coping skills, and although I was scared to death on so many levels, we would move forward in search of happiness and contentment. The financial stress that comes with life, and life with a chronic medical condition, is never ending.

As for navigating an adult, romantic relationship, I need and require respect, common interests, open communication and an understanding of what simple things in life mean. It really is that simple, and I seek it in all my relationships. I've been described as an enigma and far too independent when it comes to my intimate relationships. I am single as of today, and for the most part I prefer it that way. I have my dog, and a dog will love you when you can't stand yourself. Unconditionally!! My happiness is mine to make, even with chronic disease in the realm.

The Big Move

NOT LONG AFTER that chapter of my life, I began to investigate a move to start anew and see where my research on medical treatments would take me. My first place of interest was North Carolina, as it was home to Wake Forrest, who were doing stem cell research. Stem cells REALLY sparked my interest. During the Thanksgiving break of 1999, Hillary and I took a road trip! It was a decent week. A lot of driving, and for me, I wasn't comfortable, so it just didn't sit right. I wasn't going to take it as a defeat, just a delay.

After the emotionally charged episodes and my deteriorating health of the past few years, the toll it was taking on my body, and being advised, yet again, to "put your affairs in order," something had to change. How great it would have been if I had been able to have a few affairs of my own? I say this with sarcasm. With my usual attitude and the help of my mom and brother-in-law we put a few safety nets in place to protect and support Hillary in the event of my demise. I spoke in depth with my physician and he did agree that the weather of a drier, warmer climate may help to ease some of the body pain and make my remaining time a bit easier to deal with. Letters were written and steps were taken to make this happen.

Another court appearance with the ex would take place so that custody issues, child support, etc. could be addressed. Up until this point, he had blown off visitation, wasn't paying child support, or carrying health insurance. I was given the permission by the court to move, with Hillary, to Arizona. Wayne laid the ground work and finalization himself based on his lack of actions to this point, for the move to go forward. Again, he would call and make waves on occasion, blame me for everything, etc., but at this stage and based on her age, it was the court which ordered it to be Hillary's call as to if she wanted to see and/or be with her father. Mind you, she flew east every summer after our move west, often for a month, and sometimes longer, and spent time with both sides of the family until she graduated from high school. Her desire to interact with her father was not my call, it was just NOT part of her plan. She had her own reasons, and it was important that those individuals involved understood that. I believe to this day they completely understood this, even if at times they had hoped for change. After all, there is always hope, but often, in my experience anyway, it is best to let go and move ahead with life and often it is not without emotional pain or heartache, but hopefully with a lesson learned.

After all the legalities of my side were handled, my parents and I merged two households and headed west with no real plan, just a welcoming change of lifestyle.

The trip west with my parents took us about a week driving across the country and making a few stops along the way. We stopped strategically across the country to say good-bye and visit with certain family members with whom we were close, and lived outside of Massachusetts. We arrived in Arizona in July of 2000.

To say this was a cultural change was an understatement. People have often described me as laid back and slow when I lived in Massachusetts, but this took that description to an entirely different level. Looking back, it had a lot to do with the landscape. In New England, streets are often lined with heavy foliage making visuals regarding distance limited, unless you were up in the mountains of Maine, Vermont, or New Hampshire. Out here in Arizona, once you leave the desert floor, which is pretty flat, and head to the higher desert, the views or scenic vistas are breathtaking. Sunsets and sunrises are so majestically beautiful. On the east coast I only recall seeing these sights on the coastline of Cape Cod or Maine.

We settled into our new home, a new mobile home not far from my aunt (mom's younger sister) and uncle. This was part of the plan of us landing in Arizona, that my mother and her sister could be close for the first time in many, many years as they aged, or as my mom would say "together for their twilight." The dry heat also made my father a bit more mobile, thus a tad happier. We had a new small family unit for which we would do and see many new things. I was not working, having started collecting disability in 1999 after 2 ½ years of having to prove declining health. It was exciting and frightening at the same time, but we had a fresh start in a new place. It was my health that at the time seemed to be the main concern and that would change rapidly upon our arrival.

We were not in Arizona more than a couple of months and we had a lot of company. MJ and his family came to visit for a couple of days in August of that first year, a brother-in-law with family in Phoenix came to visit in October. They were really great visits with a little sight seeing tossed in. The following spring, a cousin and her husband came to visit. It was fun to see those we spent so much time with on the east coast and show them around some of the nearby attractions of our new homeland.

It was not long after our arrival in Arizona when my parent's health began to decline considerably, and rather quickly. Upon our arrival we had waiting in the mail a letter telling us that my father was in immediate need of medical attention to address heart issues which had landed him in the hospital back in Concord, MA just prior to our leaving the area. At the time, HMOs were the norm and given his age, it was our conclusion that the medical system did not want to address those issues in Massachusetts. So our initiation into the medical facilities of Arizona, and the Phoenix area were about to become ritual. Dad's issues were addressed and he began to recoup. My mother had a long history of heart disease and high blood pressure along with a couple of TIAs dating back a number of years prior to our move to Arizona. Those would become more and more of an issue as time went by. She would suffer a couple of heart attacks, a major one resulting in by-pass surgery. Follow-up carotid artery stents were eventually placed which resulted in a stroke and a diagnosis of Parkinson's disease. I learned my way around Phoenix pretty quick in the first three years alone.

I knew upon our arrival in the small Arizona town we decided to settle in that the medical services in the area were minimal, especially in the specialty department. I had always had access to top notch doctors and hospitals in the Boston area, and, given the long-term diabetes and the family history, a decent doctor was on the top of my to-do list. There was not one endocrinologist within a hundred miles, meaning I needed to find a doctor that could and would treat me. Locating doctors for all of us was a priority pretty much right out of the gate. I had enough supplies for my insulin pump, glucose strips and lancets, etc., to last three months, giving me a bit of time to shop. With my parents having undergone heart procedures almost immediately upon arrival, I hooked up with a local cardiologist associated with a big heart hospital in Phoenix. It was a start. He was acceptable with the exception of his snide remarks made in my records regarding "having everything done but an autopsy" and the living situation with my parents, noted as the "mental rental." Really?! Is this sort of crap documentation really called for in a medical record? This doctor would die within five years. As time went on, I learned a lot of what should, and should not be of relevance in any given situation. I found myself always on the internet investigating a medication, a diagnosis, a treatment procedure, and/or alternative treatments for both my parents and myself. I was always reading as I often couldn't sleep, and this lit up my interest in science and medicine.

In those first four years, my mom had done maybe 6-8 stays in a Phoenix hospital, my father three. Phoenix was a 2.5-hour ride from our home at the time. Oh, I would totally take care of my mother with no qualms or complaints as she had a brain and understood what was involved. My father … was an entirely different breed. He was worse than a kid when it came to medical care. I recall while having his legs stented and having to stay over-night inpatient, he was all worked up stating he saw people watching him through a picture on the wall. Now, don't get me wrong, I can totally relate to the anxiety that accompanies medical procedures, maybe that is why I choose to do mine alone, on my own. This visit turned into three days to include pre-op, treatment, and recuperation. Money was pretty tight and so staying in a hotel was out of the question for me. Mom stayed back in Chino Valley not knowing her way around the Phoenix metro area, and so that Hillary wouldn't miss school. It was decided that I would go with Dad. Mom really wasn't driving much anymore and city traffic wigged her out. First day was okay as he could go out with me prior to admission. The night of treatment was pure and total hell for me. Completely exhausting, like a bad episode of the "Twilight Zone." He couldn't and/or didn't respond so great to morphine. He was freaking out with the aliens and others spying on us through that photo on the wall. This went on for hours while I was trying to sleep in a pull-out chair-bed. Exhaustion setting in I decided I was going to call and introduce myself to Massachusetts brother-in-law's older brother and his wife. I made the phone call to Pam. "Hi, this is Binky. I know you don't know me, but I am sure you've heard a lot about me." With that phone call a friendship of infinite proportion had been forged with her and her husband, Jim. They invited me to dinner where we talked about all kinds of things, and they even invited me to spend the night. I declined on that initial invitation, but now had a place to call a retreat in the future for medical trips that were about to come about, and they would become frequent as time went on.

Along with these medical crises would come the calls back east to my brothers to inform of any given situation status. I had always thought in my mind that as our parents aged we would become closer as siblings. Oh man, was I wrong on that delusion. It seemed that with each passing medical event in which doctors on this end would say "serious" or "critical" came the question, do they come, do they not come? In all reality, this was not my call, but with my mother's request that I tell my brothers, I did what was asked, thinking to some degree that a support net was out there. I felt so stretched at times.

The messenger always takes the heat, or so it seemed. I needed to give them this option not only to keep my conscience clear, but to allow them to make and/or address any of their own issues regarding any given situation and/or what may derive from it. I recall my oldest brother making a statement at one time regarding my mother's "last" hospital stay that he had already made two trips out prior and she wasn't dead yet. This sort of comment didn't sit so well with me but, again, not my problem. I was doing what I needed to do and that was caring for my parents, caring for myself, tending to Hillary and her needs, and the outside world had to cope with their own choices. This sort of emotional retardation, as I call it, comes full circle in the years ahead. In my experience I often feel it is a male mentality, a denial of sorts, so that THEY can cope, regardless of who they shit on in the process.

In **2002**, I finally had a decent PCP and he would care for me up until his death in 2005. I was devastated at losing him to his own demons of suicide upon returning from a summer trip east. I really enjoyed the level of communication we had. He respected my knowledge of my own disease and my body on said disease. He was a kidney specialist and was also taking care of my mom's renal issues at the time. Day-to-day life moved along. Hillary seemed to be involved and engaged at school with band, sports, and making a few friends. She has never made friends easily due to trust issues.

In **2004** I underwent a partial hysterectomy due to uterine fibroids. I asked my PCP if I would see him while I was inpatient and he stated "only if there is a problem." Imagine my surprise when he showed up at the foot of my bed the day after surgery. "What are you doing here?" He replied with, "They have a problem." I asked what the problem was and his response was that the nurses had no idea how to deal with my insulin pump. His notes clearly stated "patient can handle her own insulin requirements." When I asked why they called him, he said his presence was requested even though he told the staff I was more than capable, maybe even more than himself, to handle my insulin pump. He laughed, did a quick assessment, and reinstructed the nursing staff to allow me to handle my own insulin needs. Needless to say, it turned into five days of instructing each nursing shift of how to operate and what was involved in my insulin pump therapy. Honestly, I was a bit perplexed at the lack of knowledge. Surgery went well until a few days after discharge. Recovery was 4-6 weeks and after a week at home, I was taken back to the hospital via ambulance with a wildly irregular heartbeat which was chocked up to anesthesia reaction of sorts. This would become an ongoing situation in which over the next three years I would be on various medications and undergo multiple surgeries and procedures.

In this same time-frame from 2002 to 2005 I would undergo, 3 pulmonary vein/cardiac ablations to correct the irregular rhythm, a laser surgery to address a bout of HPV/severe cervical dysplasia (a cancer precursor) and a 6-week run of topical chemotherapy to treat the same diagnosis, and a 5-day inpatient detox to get me off of Vicodin which had been prescribed as a method of treating fibromyalgia (diagnosed in 1995) and joint issues. I was seeing a PCP, an endocrinologist, a gynecologist, a gynecological oncologist, a neurologist, and a cardiologist at the time. That, in and of itself, was exhausting both physically and emotionally. In spite of all the medical happenings, I still wanted a life that resembled a sense of normal.

Going Back to School

IN THE FALL of **2004,** I had decided to go back to school. I figured my body may not be playing nice with life, but I still had a brain and an overabundance of personal medical experience to draw on. I had spent years researching and reading anything and everything that was coming down the pike regarding Type 1 diabetes, along with all the research I had been doing over the past few years regarding my mother's health issues. I concluded that I should put it to some money-making use. Not only that, but I really needed some personal stimulation outside of the household. I enrolled in the local community college program to become a medical transcriptionist. I was really enjoying the classes and met some really wonderful people along the way. I also met some pretty arrogant individuals. You know those types that seem to know it all already and did not hesitate to offer up their cures for me. I often thought to myself, "Why are you wasting your money on college classes when you already know everything?" As I have often told Hillary over the years, it doesn't matter where you go, or what you do in life, work, or personal, you are going to encounter these types of individuals. I would often let their crap roll down hill and over my need or use for them, but, then there were times I just couldn't take it anymore and would throw verbal word vomit at them in the form of a one-lined zinger. "Really, you think the God at your church can cure me?" "I'll pass; if God wanted me cured, he would have done it by now." People are always mistaking Type 1 for Type 2 diabetes. I still find this to be a complete and total ignorance on the part of people who claim they know many people who have been "cured." Again, Type 1 individuals produce NO insulin. Type 1 is an autoimmune response. The only treatment is insulin, via injections or an insulin pump. This has been the way since the beginning of knowledge on the disease in the early 1900s when insulin was discovered. No insulin, no life!! Type 2 diabetes, sure, you can cure it, or put it into remission with diet, exercise and/or oral medications, and insulin. Type 2 is a lack of the body's' ability to utilize the insulin it produces, creating what is know as insulin resistance. Type 2s who don't follow these protocols often find themselves losing a limb, or in organ failure much faster than a Type 1.

My theory on this is that by the time many people with Type 2 are diagnosed it has been in an active disease process for many years. Also, those who find themselves facing this diagnosis often face denial, depression, and a lack of wanting to change their habits and behaviors which only leads to more complications and a longer period of time in which those complications are worsening to the point of no return. At the age of 9-years, I, too, had the denial, the anger and an outright 'fuck this' attitude.

I have known since early childhood what my risks were associated with the disease. I totally pushed the envelope with my early life choices and always with that line hanging in the back of my head. "She'll never see 21." I saw 21 come and go. My only successful pregnancy to term at the age of 25 brought the arrival of Hillary. I was well aware of what that process could possibly result in. I was told as a teenager that having children was probably not in my best interest. I remember the movie "Steel Magnolias" coming out in the fall I was pregnant with her. Little did many know, I had read the book, so I knew the end result was death. It was not something I was going to think about. Pregnancy was a lot of work and I was not always successful in staying one step ahead of the possible complications and had no real spousal support. It was after the birth in 1989, along with the marital chaos and the drama of those involved in much of it, that problems were beginning to make themselves front and center. The gut issues ultimately diagnosed in 1995-97 would be a major complication which made any sort of blood sugar control impossible.

While my parents continued with their own health dilemmas, I too, was living and dealing with my own issues. You see, people often don't understand that stress eludes no one. This holds true for me as well. I have never thought I used my disease as an excuse, but there did come a time I needed to learn to say no to others because I knew my body was not going to allow anything else. It can be incredibly frustrating when one really wants to take part in life's activities and your body, for any given reason, just will not allow you that joy. I was, and remain, thankful for my humorous outlook on any given situation, even those that are dark and painful.

While taking classes it was a challenge, but worth every minute. It was supposed to be an 18-month program. It took me two years due to the heart surgeries and one gynecological surgery. The chemo had been penciled in over the summer while I was on break and Hillary was visiting back east. Hillary and I were no longer cohabitating with my folks. My mom was always just a phone call away for moral support. I was so grateful for our open conversations about topics that would make some squirm. She was often just a calming comfort. Her comfort though in an active medical situation going back many years would have me doing much of it on my own. I know she was just being a mom who didn't want to see her baby hurting in any form. For me, (I've applied this thought process to others for whom I have "been there" to support in a medical situation) to be of real help is to remain calm. There were times when I was being poked beyond reality and my mother would get upset and start snapping at the nurses. Now, don't get me wrong, there were several who really needed that bark for the attitude of "I've been doing this for X number of years." That didn't mean shit to me when they couldn't locate a vein after 6 or 8 pokes. I have never had good veins, but as the disease process goes on, the veins tend to get smaller, thus, I am now afflicted with small vessel disease. I have held up my share of operating rooms and procedures, and lab techs, due to the fact many often can't get access with a line. In the past 25 years or so, it has just been one affliction after another. I really have no choice but to take the ride and be as happy as I possibly can while on it. I know there are times when friends get tired of hearing me cancel plans, but that is my reality. The stress on my body and my emotional well-being have become what I need to address for myself. No one else can do this for me, as they reap any ill effects of my saying yes to any and all. I know where my priorities should be and that is all that matters to me as sleeping at night is one of my favorite outlets.

Trail of Great Loss
2006 – 2008

THIS TIME IN my life I swear I was on autopilot most days. There was the certain amount of ritual in caring for myself and tending to the needs of my parents. Up early, shower, off to work. Hillary was a junior/senior in high school and doing all that college prep stuff, her band activities, prom and an upcoming surgery of her own. In 2006 she was back on the east coast for the summer. I, too, had flown back for a two week vacation which included the graduation of two of my nephews. I stayed with my oldest brother and his family, his oldest son being one of the graduates. We had an awesome visit. I also knew that a very special lady, a woman Hillary referred to as "Grammie" had not been well and her time was limited at best. Well, we didn't get the opportunity to say goodbye as she had passed away the morning we arrived in Boston. Not the best way to start a vacation, but we continued with the visiting and reminiscing of a wonderful woman and a fabulous legacy of the boys she raised to be out of this world men. Grammie was the mother of my brother-in-law (by marriage), Mark and his brother, Jim, for whom I have become the sister he never wanted. Graduation ceremonies took place, parties followed, and Hillary and I got to see a lot of people we hadn't seen since leaving MA for AZ, six years prior. I would fly back to AZ and Hillary remained on Cape Cod with E's family. She would spend at least a week or two with them every summer, along with a week or two with family on her dad's side. I was home and back to work when I got a phone call one afternoon from Pam, "Mark's gone." I had a major meltdown, completely lost it. I was hysterical crying. I could not comprehend this call. She told me to process and she would call me back later. A million thoughts ran through my mind. NO! Why? How?

Hillary was now alone on the Cape with her cousin. I had to rid my body and mind of the tears before I could go forward. I was numb, as was his wife and children and many others. You see, I had just spent several days with Mark and family at their home. We had a wonderful trip up the Maine coast, even in the rain, attended his youngest daughter's graduation from kindergarten, and he had taken me to the airport for my return flight to Arizona. With the exception of the visible grief of having just lost his mom, and his older brother several months prior, he seemed okay health-wise. He had suffered a massive heart attack. He was only 44-years-old, which is far too young, and his loss was felt by many. I know Hillary felt, as did I, a gaping hole in our hearts as we were very close to Mark. Since our move to Arizona, Mark's brother, Jim, and I have been through enormous challenges over these past years. Jim, is always there for me. I joke that I am the sister he never wanted. A ticket back to Boston was booked and I flew back to console and support Hillary and attend services. Not that I needed a reason, or an excuse, he was a huge influence in the upbringing of our Hillary. He called her his "pseudo-daughter" and to this day, he holds a very special place in our hearts.

Upon my return to Arizona, Hillary staying behind for another month, my mother had a deep chat with me about death, dying, and whether planned and expected or sudden, it is always difficult. BUT ... I hated those "buts" in our conversations, she continued by stating to me that she hoped when she crossed over that I would not react as I did on this unexpected passing. I was sort of in shock as it was sudden and unexpected. I had just been with him and he seemed fine, other than his own deep and current grief. He was far too young to go so soon, and so suddenly. Time moves on for those left behind, but that hole of a lost loved one rarely heals completely.

A year goes by and in July 2007, a couple of weeks after Hillary graduates from high school, her father dies of renal cancer. Hillary had just started a new job as a CNA in training, a requirement for her nursing degree. She questioned as to whether or not she wanted to fly to Boston for services. I told her that it was her decision, and either way, I would support her. I, however, would not be returning to the east coast for his services.

Why would I? All I saw in that venture was a lot of resentment, unnecessary tension, and a lot of drama and bullshit that I didn't need to deal with. I placed that old adage, "a time and a place" and this was not it knowing full well how a couple of his sisters felt about me, like him, always blaming someone else. Hillary decided for reasons of her own that she would return for her father's services. She borrows the funds to fly back as money was not in abundance for travel. Hillary had her own emotional issues she wanted to deal with regarding her father, and I understood that completely. I did feel a bit like I was tossing the lamb to the lions, but I knew there would be at least a handful of direct paternal family members that would be in attendance to support her and others who would be at her side at the drop of a dime. All I will say here is my daughter came back totally appalled at some of the comments made by people who stated things like "Oh, gee, we didn't know he had another daughter." Yep, to those who were always singing his praises for the love of his daughter, maybe you should ask her about the undying devotion that lacked on his part. In any event, she did what she had to do on her own terms for her to deal and heal. She made this trip for her own well-being; all I could do is support her emotionally as I always have. My mother, on the other hand, was giving me the business about my attitude. Why? Why would I go back for that? Why would I place myself in that toxic type of situation? I had put most of my issues with him behind me with the exception of his treatment towards our daughter, his own flesh and blood, for whom he never treated as anything more than an irritation, an inconvenience, a pawn. I'm sorry, no love lost there. Honestly, given some of the things he put in his body over the 17 years we were together, and the really stupid acts that could stem from that inges- tion, I am surprised it took as long as it did. He was 47 years old.

Along with his death came a wave of mixed emotions. I had spent SO many years, young impressionable years, with this man who in the big picture of life, I don't believe ever really loved me, or if he was even capable of such emotions as love. That being said, I had and continue to hold many fond memories of my time with many of his family members.

We move forward six months to November 2007. My Uncle John passes away shortly after undergoing a risky heart procedure to try and extend his declining heath. He had been the Air Force recruiter who enlisted every one of my older brothers. It had been a tense, touch and go few weeks after his surgery. He had come down with C-diff infection and never quite got over it. We had taken part in so many outings with him and my Aunt Martha (my mom's little sis- ter) since our move to Arizona. He was nonstop, always going, al- ways doing something productive. He was a very skilled individual in many aspects. He was always a gentle soul where I was concerned. Always even tempered, unless we were "debating." He had crossed over less than ten minutes after Hillary and I had left the hospice, my mother telling us the news upon our return to Prescott from Phoenix. Upon entering their apartment, it was visible that my parents were in a deep, deep state of grief, and rightly so. My mother had nothing but praise for Uncle John, always being there when she needed some- thing, from the time of their early days of marriage, and when their children were all small. There was a long history between them all.

The loss of Uncle John in November took a deep toll on my sweet and always dear Aunt, who was my mother's youngest and only sister. She was beside herself in grief, and began to drop noticeable weight for which we had all associated with her emotional status, not eating as much in her grief. It's not uncommon. Unlike my parents, my aunt and uncle did everything together. Always where there was one, the other was close by. It was almost six months to the day, in May 2008, we lost Aunt Martha as well. She had been on a vacation in Florida visiting old friends and became ill. She flew home, was admitted to the hospital, diagnosed with lymphoma and died two weeks later. I was heartbroken. I had, at her request, been with her for a lot of the testing while she was in the hospital, until they moved her to hospice. I loved her deeply and know she loved me as well. We certainly had our share of laughs and inside jokes. The passing of these two exceptional individuals and the time we had all spent together since our move to Arizona was unbelievable. Like a hole had been ripped out of my world. As a child in Massachusetts, when they lived in nearby Connecticut, I would often spend a week during the summer at their home. There was always an adventure, always learning and seeing something new. My Aunt Martha was incredibly gifted, talented in art and music, and I always believed she should shout that from the roof top and share her talents. She seemed to be very "shy," for lack of a better term, in boasting about her own skills and accomplishments. I hold many, many fond memories of our times together, good or bad, regardless of circumstances. To this day I display several treasured pieces of art that she created for me over the years. They light my home with her spirit.

My Biggest Loss

MY MOTHER'S HEALTH already in deep decline, fell into a deep depression after the loss of her little sister. She had always seen herself going first. Mom had not had the best recovery from her coronary bypass surgery in 2006, having come down with the C-diff infection which nearly killed her at that time. The Parkinson's was advancing much faster since this surgery as well as having suffered a small stroke after having stents placed in her carotid arteries. The loss of her younger sister was more than she could bear, her heart was clearly broken. She had told me many times that she was prepared to go first, always. With this loss of her sister, and life in the state that it was, she began to give up. It could be seen and felt by both Hillary and myself. My father, well, he really never saw a situation past his own nose. Everything always came back to him and how things would affect him. I know the man had feelings, but most situations revolved around what would "he" do? I will say that as my mother's health declined and her ability to get around became more difficult, he did step up. My mother indicated that they had been discussing what was to happen as they both declined with age. Again, I honestly don't think he listened, or cared much other than how he would be affected by these decisions. That fact becoming clear as my mother's time came closer to the end. He had what Hillary and I call "nervous cleaning syndrome." When he got nervous, and he clearly had no coping skills for hospitals or the happenings of or in one, he would start cleaning. So at least the apartment was always neat and tidy. He even started to do laundry, and Hillary often helped out in the big ways with him and my mom visiting between her classes, doing lunch, running errands, the occasional sleep over, etc. My mother became ill more and more frequently and in September 2008 landed back in the local hospital. She spent close to a month inpatient with them running test after test and no real answers. The doctors stated there was nothing more they could do. CW came out for a week or so and stayed with Hillary and I as he couldn't cope with my father, while mom was in the hospital and we tried to keep Dad calm. When the topic of a nursing home or assisted living was suggested as a means of keeping them together due to my mother not being able to be discharged home, my father quickly and emphatically said, "NO, I'm not going to a nursing home!" He was not moving into a nursing home, with or without her. Mom was already told she could not go home, her care would require 24/7 tending too. I couldn't do it, and Dad certainly couldn't tend to her, and she outright refused to allow Hillary or myself to alter our agenda for 24-hour caretaking. When Dad refused the suggestion of assisted living and remaining together, Mom decided she was done. Once she verbalized that decision things moved fast, too fast for me anyway. She was moved to a hospice facility, stopped all medications, and died seven days later with myself and MJ at her side.

The loss of my mother was without a doubt the most devastating loss of my life. She was my best friend, my advocate (good and bad), my mentor, my partner in warped humor. There was nothing we could not talk about. I knew she was suffering, but I was not ready for her to go, even though I think I may have given up long before had I been in her shoes. She was meticulous in her instructions to me as to what to do and how to go about doing it. I would do it all over again for her in a minute, in a heartbeat, no questions asked. It was several weeks before I actually cried over her loss. I had spent so much time in a mode of numb, autopilot existance. Go to work; stop daily at the folk's place, which was mid-point between my home and office.

I had such support from coworkers and friends. My siblings, although I know they were feeling the loss, they were not, nor had they been in the trenches for the dirty work, the day-to-day attention. Little do they know of the conversations that were held between my mother, father, Hillary and myself. Not one day has gone by since that warm fall day when my mother crossed over after I kissed her forehead and told her it was time to fly, that we would all be okay and it was okay to let go. She took her last breath while I was holding her hand and whispering my love in her ear. That is a gift that I believe only those having experienced such a relationship could ever comprehend. I wanted her here on earth, in the flesh, for my own selfish reasons and nothing more.

Her suffering was over, she was at peace, and I was forever changed.

Lost, Alone, and Running Out of Options

MY MOTHER PASSED on a beautiful fall afternoon in October 2008. It took several weeks for me to finally break down in tears. I had to go into the trunk of my car to grab something and when I popped the trunk … BOOM! There were the items which were removed from the hospice. Her pillow, some articles of clothing, a bag of CDs we used to pass the time and remain calm and inspired. I leaned in, placed my head on the pillow and completely lost my emotions. I don't recall how long I had been bawling uncontrollably in my trunk before Hillary came out and got me to come in the house. It needed to happen. I had compartmentalized any of my own feelings safely away to deal with all the legalities that come with death. Those things no one ever really prepares you for. My mother did, but they still needed to be addressed. Information for death certificates, for body donation, and all the follow-up phone calls and closures which needed to take place, with my father in tow knowing nothing, and not wanting to know because someone else was taking care of it. Why would he want to know, or put forth any effort to learn? He had Hillary and I to take care of it for him, and my mother had done it all prior to her death. He would use this mentality, for which he always did, for the next three years until he passed in August 2011.

As I tried to return to work and a sort of normal, my body was screaming with all the stress that had piled up over the past 18-months.

I have always found, at least this is my take, that I deal pretty well with life's stressful situations but my body often retaliates when the dust settles. I have been exceptionally lucky in regard to complications. I have complications that could have, and no doubt should have, taken me off the planet a long time ago. I go on autopilot and figure if it happens, it happens. I attempted to refocus on my new career as a medical coder, but demanding childlike requests from my father would begin to take their toll on the entire family unit. Hillary was the ultimate God-send at this time. She seemed to be the only person Dad really listened too and she told him in no uncertain terms on most occasions that we could only be doing the rituals at scheduled times. He was very petty and self-centered, always.

Stem Cell Mission

IN JULY 2009, my first birthday without my beloved mother, I found myself working, automatically tending to my father, and spending every evening for hours on the internet researching what to do about my own declining health. It wasn't as if I had neglected my own health status, but in a way seemed I had put others ahead of myself for a long time now. Hillary was in nursing school and I had been studying to take the coding certification exam for which I was scheduled the week after Mom had passed. Needless to say, I flunked! I went back to the study books and tried again 3 months later, successfully passing the exam. In my research and trolling of the internet late into the night I came across a clinical trial for islet cell transplantation. Destruction of the Islets are the main culprit to the Type 1 diagnosis. The killing off of these cells by one's own immune system triggers the disease. I was intrigued, read and investigated the process, what was involved, what could potentially happen, and the goal of outcome. They had been performing these surgeries for a few years with pretty good success. With no reservations, I sent off my name for information on how to participate in the trial. That was how I celebrated my 45th birthday; without my mother to discuss this venture with, her spirit being felt within me a new passion was born.

I remember the looks on the faces of a couple of coworkers when I returned to work the next day and made the nonchalant announcement of how I had inquired about taking part in this transplant trial and what it would entail. I had no real fear, only excitement for what life could be like. The facial expressions of a couple, said otherwise. After all, they had been witness to more than a few episodes of "stupid" (a term we use to describe a low blood sugar) and a couple of others involving pump malfunction, and my nasty mood and physical changes that can often accompany these situations. It is often not a pretty sight.

Time went by and I filled out a ton of paperwork, had numerous phone conversations with the trial coordinator, and spoke to my attending physicians to finally get the go ahead, the medical blessing. Although treatment costs would be covered by the trial, the travel to and from San Francisco, would cost money, a lot of money, for which I didn't have. My friends and coworkers kicked into overdrive with fundraising efforts, newspaper articles, yard sales, raffles, etc. were set into motion. I was feeling the love! This was a six-month process. The time came where I was scheduled for my "virgin voyage" to San Francisco, California for a weeks' worth of testing to see if I would qualify on the medical front to undergo the transplant. This was the last leg of the application process. If I passed all the testing, I was in!

Deborah Schultz, AKA Deb-Deb, a coworker friend, was the surefire travel partner to accompany me on this journey as Hillary had nursing classes for which she could not yet miss this much time. She stayed home with our dog, Maggie, who was just a pup, and her own set of anxiety and thoughts on this adventure. Deb-Deb and I loaded the car and off to San Francisco we headed. It was like the great unknown. This trip took place in March 2010.

Now, up until this point, Deb and I were friendly on the coworker front, but our outside work relationship had really just begun. As my mom's days neared an end, Deb and I had become quietly closer. That was about to change! She arrived at my home early on a Saturday morning for our departure to the pacific coast for my Monday morning admission to the UCSF hospital campus. We were all prepared with snacks, beverages, GPS bitch, and a can of Febreze. We drove 13 hours, with an occasional stop to use the bathroom and have a bite to eat. As we approached the Bay Bridge that evening, we realized we never even turned on the radio! Her version of this adventure is told on the following pages, but we talked the entire trip, and in a Toyota Corolla! Not one moment of that trip would I change. It was a milestone, another life changing moment for this girl.

At this point in the process I had started a blog that would describe all I was going through, how normal life takes a toll on the body as a long-term Type 1, informational articles and outlets for such. I had a decent following for a while, and although I have not posted in some time, it continues to get hits. This outlet was an incredible source of encouragement and support leading up to this virgin voyage.

http://et63-hope-thetransplantjourney.blogspot.com/

It was a week of ups and downs for me. I spent three days inpatient at UCSF to undergo a myriad of testing for which I had to be under medical supervision and for the documentation purposes of the study. A couple of these tests had me feeling like death was right outside the door, so I really was comforted by the medical supervision. The staff was amazing, and although there were a couple of scary moments, I felt safe in the knowledge and expertise around me. Everything was going well and being stated as such. I would be a great candidate. They discharged on the third day and all we were waiting on was one blood test that had to be sent to Washington, DC for processing. The infamous PRA (protein reactive antibody) result was what I needed to wait on for acceptance and this would take a couple of weeks.

Deb and I spent the next couple of days doing the tourist thing around the Bay area and I had a freaking blast even though my body was feeling otherwise. We did lunch in China town, walked the pier and enjoyed some amazing seafood, fabulous shops, and several people encounters for which we would both be laughing about for years to come. I have such fond memories of this trip and the friendship that has grown from it. I am, and will be, forever grateful to this woman for her continued love, support, acceptance and encouragement, as well as the endless laughing we seem to do when we are in others' company.

Upon our arrival home, Deb transferred her belongings to her vehicle and home she went.

Always Something

I DECIDED TO unpack and call my Dad. No answer. I allowed some more time to pass and called again. No answer. Well, this was bizarre as I couldn't figure out where he could be. I made a call to my cousin for whom I thought he may be with. Not there. I called Hillary, who was at work at the hospital to let her know I was home safe, and if she had any clue as to where her grandfather may be. Nothing. I was growing increasingly concerned. I had purchased a large quantity of saltwater taffy on Pier 39 and wanted to bring it to him and tell him about the trip. He never really understood the disease, the process, or the things that could and did happen anyway, but I did like to attempt to keep him in the loop. I put Maggie in the car and off we went with taffy in tow. We got to the apartment, and for some reason my gut sank. When I arrived in the parking lot, his car was parked in his spot. So, where was he? I unlocked the door and let the dog go in first. She ran in circles, sniffed high and low, and went into the bedroom, no dad. Now I am really getting freaked out. I called Hillary back and asked her to check the hospital ER to see if he was there. Nope, he was not there. I returned home and continued to call the house every hour or so throughout the night.

At 5 o'clock the next morning I got a call from the ICU unit at the hospital, "We have your father here."

Well, WTF! Hillary had checked the ER, no one had him on record. She worked on the 4th floor, no record of him there either. He apparently had suffered a heart attack and called the ambulance on his own. When arriving at the ER he told staff NOT to call his grand-daughter and that I was out of town. It was pretty serious and the call was eventually made to us. Off to the hospital we went. This incident would exacerbate the caretaking regarding my father. I was listed as healthcare power of attorney with Hillary as back up for both of my parents. At some point they HAD to call us. I was so irritated, yet relieved we now knew where he was. Again, I got no reprieve in bouncing back from my week of testing.

The next couple of weeks passed and one afternoon while in my boss' office for a meeting my phone rang. I looked at my phone and my heart sank, it was the call I had been waiting for. I asked if I could please take the call and removed myself from the meeting. I couldn't get my breath in anticipation of results. It was not the news I had hoped for. The PRA test, that was sent to Washington, had come back at a level too high and for which I would be disqualified from the trial process. The value of the test needed to be 50 or less, and mine returned at 63. I didn't know if I wanted to puke or cry. I was told that these were NIH regulations/guidelines for the trial and they could not be fudged. I was told that this result of 63 would mean that I would wait much longer for a cadaver donor match, and that I risked a higher rate of rejection.

To say I was devastated, was an understatement.

In the weeks that followed this call I fell into a state of depression. What would I do? How can I keep up a good fight given my current status? I wanted better, I wanted to live, I wanted to experience, if only for a short time, what it would be like to be normal. I wanted a cure and I wanted to play some sort of role in that cure. It was not meant to be.

Re-think – Re-evaluate

I CONTINUED TO go to work, engage while there, tend to my father and continue to support Hillary in her education and life as we knew it. Dad was recovered from the March heart episode, yet continued to decline with the effects of vascular dementia. This was not in the least bit amusing or easy to cope with. My brothers seemed to think that because Dad knew who they were when they decided to call, which was not all that often, was proof all is well. It became imperative that we take the car away from him. As in take away the keys and remove it from the easy accessibility of the parking lot. It was moved to our driveway. Dad was not the least bit happy about this, and let me know at every opportunity he got. I'm sorry, but it is my opinion that our responsibility is to step in when our aging parents are no longer capable of making safe decisions. He would continue to try and coerce doctors, especially the cardiologist, to make me give him his car back. "I'm okay to drive." Aaarrrgggg!!!

This day in and day out bullshit was so wearing and exhausting on one's soul. It was a major suck of energy and emotion. Yes, he was my father, but my five siblings, a couple of them more than others would just say "I'm not doing it, he was always an asshole to us." It got to the point where I just wanted to wipe my feet of all of them and be done. I would talk to the air (my mother and God) and ask for guidance. Every time I did this in the beginning, all I heard was her voice stating as she did a few times in life, "He's not my problem anymore." I so completely got this now and she was so deserving of that peace. I now understood her questioning of my siblings' behaviors as well in her final few years.

I would begin, in the midst of my depressive state, to deepen my research on the usage of stem cells. On the nights I found I couldn't sleep, and that became a regular occurrence, I was in deep amazement of the things I stumbled upon. Other areas for which I had followed in the past and lost track of, were alive and well in the research arena and I wanted a piece of it.

Taking a Leap of Faith

AFTER A FEW weeks of getting back to the daily grind at work and trying not to focus too deeply on the "what ifs," I began reading and researching again into alternative treatments and therapies. This was not an easy task given I felt so incredibly deflated, defeated. When the depression lifted from the disappointment of rejection from the islet cell trial and attempting to maintain health status given the erratic blood sugar patterns that had gotten me to this point; I began to think of it as fate. It was not in my cards to take antirejection drugs. Anything that requires antirejection drugs, in my opinion, is not a cure. It is merely a means of buying some quality time, and that is if there are no ill side effects from said drugs. That still remains a deep hope for many. Those drug cocktails can do damage, and research has proven that over time most transplants will give out. A heart, a liver, or kidney, if a patient can hold onto the transplant in the early phase, after 5 – 10 years of being on antirejection drugs, will require another, if you are lucky. This was a topic in which the doctors stated while undergoing my initial screenings for the islet trial. To all those who have survived much longer and with no real issues, my continued best to you as you are amazing! These people are my inspiration. They are pioneers! I have followed several personal stories which revolve around many aspects involving the "Hope for a Cure." I believe there is a genetic contribution, a chemical makeup on a lot of levels in that some people can tolerate those sorts of medications better than others. I also believe that we all make choices in our own healthcare, or we should. For me quality vs. quantity of life, and what will be best for myself as an individual. In hindsight, I do believe that cell transplant rejection, trial or not, was fate for me and was not in my best interest, no matter what the outcome.

My focus was drawn deeper to the stem cell arena, and with this determination I plowed forward with much enthusiasm. I was at a point where I fully felt I had nothing to lose, and everything to gain. The research, science, and medicine involved are mind blowing and vast in applications. I find it so incredibly fascinating, and the vision of these scientists, researchers, and doctors must not be squashed or swept under the rug. The passion for cure and better quality of life is so evident in the doctors I have encountered who practice in this field. It is a presentation for which I am not sure I can fully describe and do these individuals the accolades they so rightly deserve.

I had read many things in regard to stem cells over the years and the potential they had to cure, regenerate, and alleviate many conditions. The more I read, the more I wanted to try this method of treatment. I spent hours, night after night, reading into the wee hours of the morning trying to gather as much information as I possibly could in regard to stem cells and Type 1 diabetes. I had read many years ago, in the 80s, an article flagged my by mother, about a scientist from Harvard, I believe, who had cured Type 1 in mice. Somehow it got squashed, swept under the rug. There was a lot of research already going on, usually in other countries, which would leave my options small at best and my eye opening realization that agencies in the United States needed some serious revamping.

I began sending emails and making phone calls, and requesting information on how to go about these treatments. Researching various companies, teaching hospitals, clinical trials, NIH, and any outlet I could find on how to get my body to become part of this new venue of science and medicine that holds so much promise for so many. The potential cure! I truly believe will involve the use of stem cells.

Based solely on my findings, I made phone calls to my final few choices. A company in Canada didn't sound legitimate, the professional knowledge I was looking for was lacking, and for which years later I would discover was fraudulent. I dodged a bullet there in going with my gut instinct. I called clinics in Germany and Russia and a facility in South America, and a company based out of California. There were some procedures/trials being done in the United States, but all seemed not yet in human trial phase or were under strict research guidelines. I wanted something I could do NOW!

After much consideration, and trying really hard to weigh pros and cons, i.e., the money involved, for which I didn't have any of it, and the travel arrangements and time commitments involved in each outlet. How would I pull this off? I had to find a means as my health was deteriorating and I could feel it. In my call to the California clinic, I was connected with the sweetest woman acting as patient advocate at the time. She was knowledgeable, personable, reassuring, and caring. We would talk off and on over the course of a few months filling out paperwork, and making arrangements to potentially undergo the treatment. I was nervous about only one thing. Where would the cash come from? To this day, insurance will not cover anything like stem cell treatments as a means of disease management for Type 1 diabetes.

I am sure that I drove my coworkers and friends nuts with all the chatter on stem cells. I would present exciting talk and everything from newspaper articles to television coverage, to data from various agencies and universities around the globe doing research. I opened up the interest window of many and before I knew it, they were jumping on to help with fundraising efforts on many levels. There was also local newspaper coverage that helped spread the word. Hillary was doing her part as well. She was in nursing school at the time and did several papers and class talks on the subject. She too, got a lot of people to realize that stem cells didn't have to include killing babies. That moral stigma associated with embryonic stem cells was rampant. She was open and on board with whatever I wanted to do to extend my life in a quality manner. After all, she had a front row seat to all that had transpired over the years.

After several fundraising events were put into motion, from a quilt raffle, large community yard sale, collection containers, and a fabulous New England Fish Fry dinner organized by friends and a local organization, along with multiple newspaper articles on the topic of stem cells and Type 1 diabetes: began to become a semi-reality. The overwhelming support I received from friends, coworkers, the community, and of course, Hillary, we were all a tad disappointed when at the end of November, I was still short a majority of the funds to pull off treatment at the end of December. What else could we do? My stamina levels were depleted and restoring that factor was nowhere in sight.

I was still working full-time, often putting in extra hours for audits and reviews. Work had its own set of players and drama always in play. One afternoon, wrapping up to go home for Christmas holiday when in came a local flower deliver person with a beautiful bouquet and a card with a generous donation for the "Cause, from Santa Claus". I still don't know who that generous gift came from, but it was still not enough to make treatment happen. When to my surprise, just after the first of the year in 2010, close friends came forward with the remaining funds and stating, "we want you to grow old with us". I was overwhelmed with emotion, and more than that, a gratitude I had never felt before. I was completely humbled by the generosity of those who just didn't want to lose me, complete strangers who showed interest in the science of stem cells and the love that was felt for me and my mission.

With securing of the funds to undergo my adipose derived stem cell treatment, final arrangements were made. In seeking the support of my endocrinologist and my neurologist, they were skeptical at best, but gave me their blessing. My primary care physician signed off on the consent. Of all my providers, I believe my neurologist had the most interest and hope for a positive outcome. A date was set, flights were booked, and the clinic took care of the rest. I would fly to Texas, as at the time of my first treatment it would be required for me to cross the border into Mexico. Again, I wasn't really worried about the treatment itself, as I was about travel into a country for which I had no knowledge of the language. NONE! French I can fake enough to get by, Spanish, not a clue. It was February 2011, and I left Phoenix in hopes of improvement with my diabetes status and my life. I had no real idea of what to expect so I was doing my best to breathe and remain open-minded and calm.

My First Treatment

UPON MY ARRIVAL in Texas I was picked up and taken to the hotel where there would be an orientation later that evening and signing of consent forms. I remember arriving to some stormy weather, high winds, and potential for rain. The smell of the ocean air blowing across my face. I found this to be a sign, a sign of cleansing and new beginnings. I was traveling alone, wearing my mother's wedding band for support, I was ready. I was remarkably calm and open to whatever was about to transpire.

Later that evening, I was sitting in the lobby of the hotel awaiting the patient advocate assigned to this trip, along with a couple of others who were also there for treatment. I can still see this lobby, myself sitting alone looking out the front doors at the windy landscape and wondering of what was to come. As I was deep in my thoughts, I noticed a very attractive, stylish woman walk across the lobby and smile at me enthusiastically, "You must be Eliza!" My first thought when I hear this line as a greeting is, "who wants to know?" To my surprise it was none other than the CEO of the clinic herself. She had her own story of stem cell treatment that was what persuaded me to go this route. I can't begin to tell you what this encounter did for my inner strength and amplified my hopes for the future of my health. I was grateful and humbled yet again.

Orientation took place, consent forms signed, and off to bed I went for it would be an early morning start, my treatment being scheduled for early the next morning and having to be fasting due to the nature of the procedure. Nothing new for me, however, I was traveling alone. That morning we all met in the lobby to be transported across the border to the clinic. I would end up riding with the clinic CEO and the US doctor who was doing the treatments at the time, and one other patient who was also traveling solo, his 2nd or 3rd treatment for his health issue. I was just a wee bit nervous at this short ride, not knowing what to expect. We managed to cross the border and landed at the clinic, which I was really surprised at the sight, not being even remotely close to anything you see here in the States. We were all greeted and treated with amazing respect and care, even with the language barrier. I remember the anesthesiologist, a beautiful woman, who spoke no English. When my turn came, I was ready. I remember laying in the recovery area and waiting on my cells to be processed and fed back to me via IV transfusion. I was coming down with something, a cold, and with the elevation changes it seemed to get worse after the sedation. I was coughing, hard, and had the couple who traveled with us that day concerned as they could hear me through the wall. Mind you, it was a folding wall made up of an accordion door. The doctor had allowed me to get up and go see my cells going through the process of activation. It was beyond my wildest dreams to see these babies coming alive and what they may do to me once reintroduced back into my system.

It wasn't long and my I.V. bag was being hung and I closed my eyes and got lost in thoughts of calming peace and the hope of a better future. I believed (I'm starting to sound like the cable guy) in this science/medicine more than I could explain to anyone in my life. While waiting for my drip to complete, I was starting to cough really hard, like an asthma attack of sorts. Doctor V. came in, checked on me, after commenting on the color coming back into my face and skin, he sent the nurse to get an antibiotic for he believed I had an upper respiratory infection. What struck me as just amazing was he paid for the medication out of his pocket, me not having any money on me. He was wonderful, excited and passionate about what he was doing, and the results that patients were seeing with these treatments.

After a long day of treatment procedures, we all headed back to the hotel on the US side. I had a bite to eat and settled in for a good nights rest as I was flying back to Phoenix the next morning. To many, this turnaround time was concerning, and on top of that I was traveling alone. I went into this procedure knowing full well anything could happen.

The next morning, with the exception of feeling winded and a little sore, I felt really good overall. I had some breakfast in the hotel café' and headed to the airport. I remember talking with a plane mate about the entire encounter and left her with info as she inquired for a loved one. This would become habit for me, talking to anyone who would listen about my stem cell experience. I was feeling almost euphoric. Upon my arrival back in Phoenix, as I stood up to collect my belongings from the overhead bin, I started to feel odd, a bit fuzzy and warm and not in a good way. It had been years since I had shown any real warning signs of a low blood sugar, so I was not positive as to what may have been going on. The unawareness of oncoming lows had become a concerning issue for my doctors. I found it a little unnerving myself. As we exited the plane, the young woman who had been sitting with me asked, "Are you okay? You look a bit dazed." I told her I was feeling a bit shaky and unsteady, that I would just check my blood sugar and call for my ride. That considerate young woman returned from the restroom to check on me again. I told her of my status. She smiled, asked again if I was sure I was okay, and went on her way.

Another act of human kindness at play.

I took the week off and returned to work to rave reviews on how I looked. That sort of surprised me, but it was a welcome benefit. I was feeling really good throughout my body. The months to come would show even more improvements, i.e., my blood sugars stabilized, my vision cleared, my pain levels were almost non-existent, and my gastroparesis, for which I had not even mentioned as an issue, was making a complete turnaround. You have no idea what a relief that was. When you spend years going day and at times a couple of weeks without moving your bowels, you notice an improvement! I am happy and overjoyed to report that today I crap on a fairly regular basis! This would be considered TMI to most people unless, you, too, suffer with gastroparesis or a slowing digestive tract. This was huge as with the slowing of your digestion makes any sort of blood sugar control close to impossible. It was a crap-shoot prior to treatment, no pun intended. Over the next few months, I considered my treatment a success.

From the Outside Looking In

IN THESE NEXT few pages I will give you a peek into my life, at me as a person, by some who know me personally, have known me in the past, present, and hopeful future. My beautiful daughter, Hillary, in her own right, has a knack for telling an impressive story, full of inflection and medical terminology that I hope engages and moves my readers as much as it did me. I refer to these entries as "From the Outside Looking In." My only wish would be that my mother, and my "other" mother could have made their contributions to this as they had insight and knowledge of me that went WAY back. Their spirit is with me always, and I firmly believe that they would be proud of the steps I have taken to advance treatment therapies for not only myself, but for countless others who suffer and struggle with Type 1 and any other autoimmune issues.

My first descriptive outlook is from a childhood friend who wrote this guest blog entry for me while I was hoping to take part in the islet cell transplant trial in 2010. Her parents, whom I have called Mom and Dad for almost 40 years, had stories in many aspects of my journey. Mom "D" especially, no doubt, had some incredible stories from over the years of my many moods, the first hand marital-addiction chaos and many joyous moments in my life. These special individuals who know the definition of unconditional love have been one of my many blessings. I am beyond blessed to have had them in my life and for the love and guidance they often gave selflessly to me.

Here we go!!

Debbie writes:

I was out, country line dancing recently with my son, his girl-friend and my daughter. We were having a good time together when Colleen, my son's girlfriend, said my son, Rick, was acting weird. I looked up to see him stumble backward as he was walking towards me like he was drunk. As he is not a drinker, I became concerned. I asked my son what was up and he said that he was low. For those of you who don't know my son, he has also been "blessed" with diabetes. He had a handful of candy and started to unwrap a piece. I looked at my son and noticed he was not really focusing in on our conversation or the questions we were asking him. His gaze was far off and it was as if he couldn't really understand us; basically because he was not really able to. When I asked him what his sugars were, he just kept saying he was low.

As we had just completed a dance where you switch partners throughout the song, I went into the bathroom and got a paper towel to wash Rick's hands. I instructed him to check his sugars with his meter. It was then that Rick focused enough to us that his meter was in the car. Stephanie, my daughter, took him outside to check his sugars. As he was leaving, Rick whispered in my ear that he forgot that he had some sugar in his car, and he sounded like he had way too many cocktails. His voice was slurred and he spoke slowly. When they re-turned, Steph told me that Rick's sugar was 56 – yikes! This was after eating a bunch of candy. For those of you who don't have or live with someone with diabetes, this is pretty low. He must have been pretty darn low before he went out to the car and it is no wonder that he was unable to focus; there was no sugar getting to his brain.

Why do I write this story? Well, the next day when I read Bink's blog, she explained what it is like when one with diabetes is low. Is this coincidence? I think not. What is different is my knowledge of being with someone with diabetes. When I hung out with Bink, I was totally in the dark. If she was to stumble backward when she was low, I probably would not have noticed. If she was mumbling or unfocused, I would have thought that she was goofing around. As Bink has mentioned, she was not really forthcoming about her diabetes, but neither was I forthcoming with finding out more information. I could say that as a teenager I was unfocused on anyone other than myself, but that would only be part of it. Another part was probably Bink's unwillingness to feel "different." As teens, nobody wants to be different. So as far as that goes, I have to respect Bink's motives of not sharing, along with my teenage self-absorbance for what they were at the time. The old saying, "if I knew then what I know now" certainly would apply for both of us, I suppose.

What is it like to have diabetes? I don't have that answer. What is it like to live with someone with diabetes? That is something I can tell you about. I would think it is frustrating, scary, tiring, and a general pain in the neck to live with diabetes. Well, guess what? It is frustrating, scary, tiring, and a general pain in the neck to live with someone with diabetes. When my son was first diagnosed, I hovered over him like a shadow. Needless to say this got old fast for both of us. He needed his space and I needed to give it to him. It was one of the hardest things I have ever had to do. I have promised my son that I would "back off" and it has been extremely arduous. I should not have promised something that I can't really follow through with. It is pretty hard to "back off" when you watch someone you love constantly live in the denial bubble. I have to stop myself from demanding that he eat an apple instead of a piece of cake. I have to stop myself from begging him to keep his sugars in control so that he won't do permanent damage to his body. I have to let go and let him be his own advocate. I must let go when I don't feel like he is advocating well. If I don't let go, that I will lose him. The kicker is, if I don't pester, I may lose him earlier than was necessary. To put it bluntly, diabetes sucks for all involved.

Now that I have played "true confessions" it leads me back to our favorite blog star – Binky, or for some Eliza – and her extraordinary upcoming adventure. Bink is willing to put herself through procedures that will not only help her out, but will ultimately help out all people with diabetes. In essence, Bink is paving the way for me to have my son around a lot longer. It is critical that we find a cure for this disease. Without brave pioneers like Bink, progress would not occur. Am I excited that Bink is going to have a healthier life? You bet your buttons. Is her procedure going to help out my own son? Well, you can bet your buttons on that too. I personally have two very important stakes in Bink's upcoming procedures. Love is a very important influence in ones life. I can say that I love that Bink is doing this for herself – unselfishly – and am proud that, in the process, she is helping all the other people in the world that have diabetes. It is because of pioneers like Bink that science can move forward in the right direction.

I am very excited with Bink's recent research that give statistics of people that have had the procedure she is going to have and have been living without diabetes for many years. I, like all of you, know that Bink's life without diabetes is going to be just as awesome! I can't even imagine what it is like waking up in the middle of the night low. I am very excited for the day that Bink just has distant memories of doing so. I am excited for the day that Bink can eat what she wants and not worry about it spiking her sugars. I am looking forward to Bink being able to go for a walk and not worry about packing an extra snack "just in case." I am also looking forward to continuing to read her blog with all the glorious updates that Bink will be writing as she experiences her "new" life without diabetes. It has been so long since the days when she has had to prick her fingers that I wonder if she will find herself doing it out of habit? I suppose Bink will be the only one to be able to answer that question, but yippie for that day!

Oh, I forgot to warn you all, but I imagine you have figured out, that I have the gift of gab. That is one of the reasons Bink and I have always gotten along so well. I better end this post as she may not want to talk to me if I continue on (and on, and on ...).

I will complete this "guest" post with an enormous thank you to the scientists that continually pursue a cure for diabetes and a big hug, kiss and undying gratitude to our friend, Bink/Eliza, for her willingness to grab the science "bull" by the horns and "ride" it all the way to a cure. Rock on my little buddy! Love ya, Deb (from MA).

Debbie's blog post was prior to the islet cell transplant trial, for which I was eventually rejected.

——⟨∞⟩——

The next outside look is from Deborah Schultz. Deb-Deb as I call her, and we have become friends that can talk for 13 hours straight with no radio! She stood by me through some very dark days with love, her own fears, and a multitude of encouragement.

Her encounters are as follows:

Eliza Tyler is my best friend in Arizona. I met her a mere ten years ago when I began working with her at our mutual place of employment. It wasn't too long after beginning work together that I had come to know of her Type 1 diabetes and that she wore a pump. Prior to knowing Eliza I had only two other past coworkers years back that I knew had this same disease. I did not, however, understand this disease process until meeting and talking with Eliza about her highs and lows and how they affected her. I have personally witnessed her highs and lows more than I care to recall over these ten years as well. A number of years ago I became concerned that if something couldn't be done for her soon that I could potentially lose my best friend to this disease. She had progressed in her disease so that she was no longer receiving those signals that she was becoming low. It could happen quite rapidly after she began driving even. It was obviously concerning her too that these warning signs she had in the past regarding a high or low was not forthcoming any longer, and she began searching for medical help to prolong her life. This is when she came upon a clinical trial in San Francisco for islet cell transplant and went after it! I quickly volunteered to make the journey with her when it was time, and I believed with my whole heart that she would be accepted into this clinical trial. I wanted my friend, as selfish as it seemed, for a long, long time. Well, eventually the time came for us to make this road trip to San Francisco for a litany of medical tests to see if she would qualify for the trial. In sum, she did not due to one lab value being outside the guidelines of acceptable according to the National Institute of Health. My friend became depressed for a time after digesting this rejection of sorts. My heart ached for her situation. There was nothing left for me to do but pray, and I did ... hard. A number of months passed and once again Eliza had researched a new medical solution. It involved using her own stem cells. The cost of this treatment was over $10, 000. All of Eliza's friends and coworkers started brainstorming what fundraisers we could handle and were once again busy little beavers in the goal of raising enough money so she could have her adipose stem cell treatment in a timely fashion. After more than a few months working hard at this goal, we were still far from seeing the light at the end of this tunnel. At that point an extremely generous monetary gift appeared, and the goal had been reached! I praised God on that day. A couple of months later in February 2010 Eliza had her stem cell treatment in Mexico. She was ill when she went for treatment with some sort of respiratory infection, but she did so nonetheless. I was so excited to see her changes and hear her describe the benefits that began happening before she even had the IV removed from her arm that contained her own stem cells. This treatment for her has been a huge success. It wasn't long and she was noticing the warning signs were there again, and she was even able to reduce the amount of insulin that she needed on a daily basis. I had even commented on her face appearing younger looking (well at least one side of her face). We laughed together about this, and still do sometimes to this day. All in all, she is better for having researched and gone through this stem cell treatment. Eliza's personality must have been shining when she went for this treatment (alone, I might add) because the founder of the organization that this treatment was performed through even asked Eliza if she would assist them in their efforts by speaking with other potential patients to answer questions regarding her experience. An outlet Eliza didn't have going into her treatment.

In December 2011 Eliza was involved in a head-on car accident during a snowstorm. As a result, she suffers with a traumatic brain injury, or TBI. While initially following the accident it was incredibly obvious that she wasn't able to track easily during conversation, and had lost her ability to respond to subtle and sarcastic humor. This was heart-wrenching to witness as this had never been an issue for her in the past, and it was obvious that her journey forward just became more complicated. Due to her TBI she ended up losing her job, her health insurance, and even her home! She kept fighting for a new sense of normalcy and has never given up hope. She underwent two additional stem cell treatments since the accident and has continued to improved each time. Today her focus is much better and while conversations aren't always fluid, she just laughs through the difficulties her new life brings her way and continues to be my best friend in Arizona.

I am so proud of Eliza. Not only has she picked herself up by her bootstraps more than a few times throughout her life, but she has fervently researched this disease for decades and is now at a point in her life where she desires to share with others her journey. She has been an infinite well of knowledge to me on this disease, and I just know in my heart of hearts that as she pours out her story in written format for others that they will laugh ~ cry ~ but they will also receive a better understanding like I have ~ and they will be touched by my dear friend as I have been.

Thank you, Eliza for paving the way for others so their journeys may be void of some of your hardships along the way.

I love you, Binky.

Deb Schultz

—◦∞◦—

Next to be heard from is my darling daughter, Hillary. She is and has been my greatest gift and accomplishment and I am SO very proud of her. You will read her input, her emotional toll and outlook on my life and disease, and what it can mean to a family member. She holds no punches in anything she does and tells it like it is, whether it is to me, her mother, or anyone else. She has become her own woman, a current Registered Nurse. Her dealings and manner of coping with me, and commentary is the following: ~~~~~

Growing up with the parent with diabetes is stressful. Will their blood sugar drop when we're in public and don't have anything to get it up? Is it going to drop in their sleep? Will they even know? Are they going to wake up in the morning? Am I going to be the one that finds them in the morning? These are all very real and scary thoughts for a child to have. I knew my mom always tried to be very aware of her sugars, but you can't be in control all of the time. At some point nature is going to do its own thing. I always felt, and still do to some extent, responsible for making sure my mom was okay. I felt like if I didn't take care of her, who would? I know now that I didn't have to take care of her, but as a teenager I always felt like I did. I suppose you could say I resented it. I mean what kid wants to worry about their mom's health when there's so much other stuff going on in life? She had both dangerously high sugars, upwards of 600, and also extreme lows, around 26, but we always got through it. There were hospital admissions and ER visits, eating binges in the middle of the night, but that was our life. Nothing about any of this ever seemed strange to me, it was just part of our life. It is something that we had to deal with all the time. It always has to be in the back of your mind. As a small child, maybe around the age of five, I was able to give my mom an injection. When I got older into high school, I used my mom for class projects, to try and explain to my classmates that it doesn't make her a different person; this is just part of our life. I remember occasionally getting upset when people would say "oh, I'm sorry" when they would find out that my mother was a diabetic. I never really understood why someone would apologize, or be empathetic to that. Maybe it was because they didn't understand. I also remember people telling my mom "if you just exercised, lost weight, you wouldn't be a diabetic, you'd be cured." That may be the case for some Type 2 diabetics, but Type 1 is a totally different form of diabetes. Type 2 diabetics, it is true that it is generally lifestyle related or that your body stops utilizing insulin the way it's supposed to, so your insulin sensitivity decreases. Type 1 diabetes is an autoimmune disorder which generally is diagnosed in early childhood to teen years, where the pancreas has stopped working completely, you produce zero insulin. My mom was diagnosed with Type 1 diabetes when she was nine years old. I remember my 9th birthday; thinking am I going to be next? Is this something that I'm going to have to live with my entire life? Is it something that my kids are going to have to deal with too? Just because your parent is a diabetic doesn't mean that you're going to be. It just means you need to be alert and watch for warning signs because you are at a higher risk for becoming diabetic in the future.

My mom has always had an exceptional outlook on life, making light of her ups and downs, and the hardships that come with her disease. I remember growing up and we never really had a lot, but she taught me to always have a sense of humor. She doesn't have any complications as far as amputations, kidney failure, having to go to dialysis, or anything like that. She does have gastroparesis, which is a slowing of digestion, the involuntary contractions of the intestine that push food through. Generally, this means decreased absorption of nutrients. When I was about 10 years old my mom was told that she didn't have much longer to live due to complications that were becoming increasingly severe. She was put on a liquid diet due to the gastroparesis. She wasn't digesting solid foods anymore. She was told to put her affairs in order. She was then put on an insulin pump. This insulin pump was a life-changer. She didn't have to take six or more shots a day anymore. She still had to check her blood sugar, sometimes in upwards of 12 times a day, but this was small compared to the repeated injections she had to take every time she wanted to eat something. The insulin pump is an implanted device, similar to an IV that you would get in the hospital. You program the amount of insulin that your body needs throughout the day to maintain, and when you eat you enter a bolus of insulin to cover the amount of food (carbohydrate) you are eating. She then started looking into stem cell research and treatment for Type 1 diabetes. I remember prior to her first stem cell treatment. One incident while we were grocery shopping. It seems to me that something about walking around a Walmart store just sucked the blood sugar from her system. She seemed fine in the store. We got all of our shopping done, got in the car and drove home, which at the time was approximately 30 minutes from the store. When we pulled into the parking spot at the apartment complex, she put the car in park, looked at me and said "we don't live here." Right then I knew. She was in "stupid mode." For years now, she's had what is called hypoglycemic unawareness. Meaning when her blood sugar drops, she no longer sees the typical warning signs. Most people who are hypoglycemic feel it. Normal symptoms would be cold, clammy skin, tremors in the hands, difficulty standing, and difficulty forming words. For as long as I can remember, my mom has been able to hold a perfect conversation with incredibly low blood sugars. Not that this is a good thing, in fact, it is quite dangerous. When a person's blood sugar drops too low they can fall into a diabetic coma, which can result in death. It's only when she stops making sense, that I know something is seriously wrong. So, when she says "we don't live here," something is serious and we need to jump on it! I told her "Come on mom we need to get upstairs." She continued to insist that this wasn't our home. So, when I finally convinced her to come upstairs, which took a little bit of work, she stood up out of the car and was immediately wobbly and unstable, similar to someone who would have had too much to drink. I managed to get her up the stairs and into the living room where I had her sit on the couch. The fastest way to get the diabetics blood sugar up is with natural easily digestible sugars. The types of sugar you find in apple juice, orange juice, and other fruits with a high sugar content. I told her she needed to drink some juice, and that I would get it for her, she just needs to sit on the couch. Well, anyone who has ever dealt with my mother knows just how stubborn she can be, so this is where it gets interesting. While she continues to sit on the couch where instructed, she proceeded to tell me "I don't want juice!" I check her blood sugar at this point, and it is a whopping 26! So, I again told her, "you have to drink the juice." As she sat on the couch the wobbling sensation caught up with her and she couldn't sit still, couldn't hold her head up straight. She kept asking me why the room was spinning. So, I again told her, "Your blood sugar is low you need to drink the juice." So, as she continues to argue with me about the juice, she hits me with this: "I don't want JUICE! I WANT COOKIES!" We had just come home with a box of Oreos. So in an effort to get her to drink the very much needed orange juice, I resorted to bargaining with her like a child. "You can have some cookies, once you drink the juice." After several minutes of bargaining, she finally agreed, and I handed her a 12-ounce glass of orange juice. She loathingly drinks the juice, which came with some really nasty looks. When the juice was gone, I handed her a stack of five Oreo cookies. Anyone who has had Oreo cookies knows that the orange juice is not an Oreo's ideal partner. So, the look of disgust on her face after she bit into that first cookie was not a pretty one. My sole goal was to get her to drink the juice, to get her blood sugar back where it needed to be. I accomplished what I needed too. Although incredibly frustrating at the time, she is still here to laugh about her unending stubbornness with me.

On the flip side of a 26-blood sugar, we have the highs. These are particularly nasty, as they are generally cause for the person experiencing them, to feel nauseated, have a headache, and if they go on for too long, they cause incredible muscle cramps, which leads to DKA, Diabetic Ketoacidosis. This too, can be life threatening if not treated.

So, one morning while I was in college, I get a phone call from my mom. She is at work, and when I answer the phone, she is incredibly grumpy. She proceeded to yell at me about not answering my phone, and so on. Knowing my mom, and that even when I bark back at her, we argue, we complain, and we eventually get over it. My response to her is "Well I answered it this time! So, what do you need?" She goes on to tell me that she changed her insulin pump set that morning, and it was not functioning correctly. She hasn't received any insulin since she got to work at 7 A.M. It is now, 11:30. So, I pack up a new pump set, her insulin and I head to her work. When I get there, a coworker of hers is standing out front waiting for me, and I am told to brace myself, she's not in a good mood. When I go in to see her, she is red in the face, her skin is hot, and she is raging pissed! I have her check her blood sugar, and low and behold, it is in the 600s. Now, this solution is clearly not as easy as a glass of OJ. To get her sugar back down within range, for her, her target is 150, she needs the appropriate amount of insulin, and time. The initial problem in this situation was that she was not receiving insulin from her pump like she should have been. This is because of what we have nicknamed "tissue issues". My mom has been a diabetic for so long, and has had to take so many insulin injections throughout her lifetime; that she now has scar tissue in most of her main injection sites, primarily, her butt, thighs, and stomach. Therefore, she has to place her pump in either an arm or an area without scar tissue, which is sometimes difficult to do. So, I get to the office, she is irate, and now her sugar has been so high, for so long, that the muscle cramping is beginning to set in. It took me and two of her coworkers to get her to the car; she was not fit to stay at work. So, we managed to get her to the car and I headed home with her. Now, my mom only worked several blocks from the area hospital, and from her office to just past the hospital, she did nothing, and I do mean nothing, but yell at me for not answering my phone, and how shitty she felt, and how her pump not functioning was "bullshit!" So, several blocks past the hospital, I slowed the car, and told her, "Do you want me to take you home and we can treat it there? Or should I turn around and I'll dump you in the ER?" She just looked me. I know, I know, kind of harsh, right? Well, sometimes, a stubborn lady needs a stubborn kid to tell her straight, this is how it's going to happen. So, she agreed to calm down, and with the exception of several moans on the ride home, did not say another word.

When we got home, we treated her by placing a new pump set in her upper arm, a series of insulin injections, and a lot of water. It seemed as though our many years of training in at home treatment was working. Until about 3 o'clock the next morning. I was awoken from a dead sleep by her moaning in pain from the other side of the house. When I got to her, she was sitting on the toilet, gagging with a trashcan between her knees. I asked her what her blood sugar was, "518." I then asked, "have you thrown up yet?" She shook her head, no. I drew up another 20 units of insulin and gave her another shot. I agreed not to take her to the hospital, said we would give the insulin an hour to work, and if she wasn't down to at least 400, or if she started vomiting before that time, we were going. I tucked her back into bed, and went to the living room to read (it was closer to her room than my bedroom). Not 15 minutes after I sat down on the couch, I heard her heaving into the trash can next to her bed. I went in to check on her, and bring her another glass of water, and tell her I was calling an ambulance. She was angry, but didn't argue, she knew it was bad. I dialed 911 from my cell phone, and the dispatcher picked up:

Dispatch: 911 how can I direct your call.

Me: Medical.

Click. Transferred call.

Dispatch: 911 what is your emergency?

Me: My name is Hillary Tyler, I live at *** Cactus Wren. My mom is a type 1 diabetic, her blood sugar has been elevated in the 4 and 5 hundreds for roughly 24 hours. She is now vomiting, diaphoretic, and I believe she is in DKA. I gave her 20 units of insulin approximately 20 minutes ago just before the vomiting started.

Dispatch: Okay, Hillary, I had an ambulance on the way. You sound like you pretty much have it under control; do you want me to stay on the line with you until the ambulance arrives?

Me: No, thank you. Please let them know, the front light is on and the front door is unlocked.

Dispatch: I will let them know. If her status changes, call us back.

Me: Thank you, I will.

The paramedics opted to wait until she was in the Emergency Room to start an IV. So, they loaded her into the ambulance. I told her I would meet her in the ER, and they were on their way. Now, a perk of knowing almost all of the hospital staff in our small town hospital due to working there, was that I was able to get more detailed updates, and they brought me back to be with her at the earliest opportunity. When I got to the ER, the front desk security and the EMT in the triage area both happened to be friends of mine. All I had to do was walk to the desk and ask. "She's in Critical Care 1." Well, shit. That's not usually a good sign. "Come on, I already told the nurse who she is. They're expecting you." Now I know that this completely sounds like she got special treatment, this is really not the case. I am just a pushy person when it comes to my family, and being a nurse, I have the knowledge to ask the right questions to get things done. So, when I got to her ER room, I sat down with her and waited for the nurse to come in. Awesome! The one ER nurse I DON'T know! However, I asked all the questions I normally would, "Did they draw blood gasses and a venous glucose?" "They did, and I'll be right in with a liter of normal saline and we'll wait on the results." I look at my mom; ask how she's feeling, although I could tell by the look on her face what the answer was going to be. A little while later, I'm not sure how long to be exact, the nurse came back in, with an insulin syringe.

Ten units of regular insulin through the IV. Direct to the circulatory system, faster acting, good call doc. Now the waiting game. So, we waited and waited. By this time, it was almost 5:30 in the morning before the doctor came in. "Her labs look okay. No DKA. Looks like you did everything you could, did everything right at home to prevent it." I asked the doctor what the values of her blood gasses were, he looked at me slightly shocked but gave me the values. Not terrible. "Sometimes, you just have to come in for an extra boost to get you back in the range you need to be in. We're going to keep you here for a little longer, just to make sure your sugar doesn't crash now, and get you better hydrated, but you'll be able to go home this morning." To that we both replied, "Thank you."

Just before shift change, about 6:30 that morning, in comes the nurse with the glucometer. Just going to check her blood sugar, and then she should be ready to go. If only it were that simple. 24! We had gone from 553 on a venous blood draw, to 24! The nurse did not believe the machine, which I admit can happen, as we are trained to use all of our senses, and evaluate the patient not the number. I looked at the nurse and told her, "It's probably accurate." The nurse then looked at me and stated, "No, I think the machine needs to be calibrated. She was holding a full conversation with you when I walked in." LADY, you don't know my mother! I told the nurse, "She can function as normal in the 20s. If you stand her up, you'll be able to tell she is low. I promise the machine is probably fine. You may want to go get some D50." But as us nurses do, she stuck with her gut, went and got a new machine, came back several minutes later, this time with the day shift nurse. This time the reading is 23. YEAH! I think it's time to get that D50 I suggested 10 minutes ago, which is exactly what they did. The nurse pushed an amp of D50, which is literally a 50% solution of dextrose, and checked her sugar several times over the next few hours. Finally, at almost 11 o'clock that morning, a full 24 hours of high blood sugars later, we headed home.

As selfish as it sounds, growing up with a parent who has diabetes makes you wonder, especially when they're told at a very young age that they're not going to live past the age of 21, if they're going to be there to see your major life events. Are they going to be there to see you go to your prom? Watch you graduate from high school or college? Or watch you get married and have kids? I have been incredibly fortunate that my mom has been around to witness most of these events. She was there to see me graduate high school and college, and she was the loudest supporter I had in the crowd for these events, and all of my high school sporting and band events. She watched me move onto a career and have my son.

Although, I am very aware of my mother's medical limitations and challenges, she works to overcome them every day. I fully expect her to be around to witness and give me away at my wedding. My mom has gone through a lot of rough times, both physical and emotional, including tissue problems, absorption problems, digestive problems, the loss of her parents, the birth of me, and a horrific car accident, that I truly feel that she can overcome any challenge she is faced with. I also know that she is going to put forth every effort she has to in order to ensure she is there for my wedding, and to watch her grandson grow as long as she possibly can. My mother is the strongest woman I know and, although she says on a fairly regular basis that she's "not sure how much longer I can do this," or how much longer she can fight, I know that she will.

Two days before my 18th birthday, I ended up taking my mom to the hospital for another round of DKA. Her blood sugar was again, over 500, from my recollection, for more than 24 hours. This time she ended up spending five days in ICU. She missed my 18th birthday, but I was there to visit every single day. She insisted that I go out with my friends and not miss the celebration. I ended up going to a hockey game with several friends and out to dinner, but I felt guilty that I was out partying with friends while my mom lay in a hospital bed. She was always really good about making sure that I didn't notice what was going on around me just because of complications of her illness. Just like when I planned to move out on my own, I felt guilty leaving her. She had told me since the time I graduated high school, "It's time for you to go out and spread your own wings." I have always known that no matter what happened, my mom didn't want me to live my life around her, and as my grandmother put it on her deathbed, "Hillary, you have to go out on your own and do what will make you happy. You can sit around here and wait for us all to die. Then what will you have left?" Her point, took me a little while to figure out. If I didn't learn to live for myself, instead of everyone else, I would be left alone, in the town that I grew up in, with nothing but old memories. No new memories made, no new experiences, no new stories. Where if I finally ventured out on my own, lived life like I was always taught to, to the absolute fullest, and like every day was my last, I could always come home. And with that, I would have new memories, experiences and stories to share with those that are still around because they will be fine. My mom has made it 38 years longer than she was told she would with a lot of obstacles, and with or without my help she is a fighter, and she is going to keep living.

Life is looking up?

CARE FOR MY father continued as Hillary worked on completing her nursing degree and I moved ahead in my position as a medical coder. I was really enjoying the challenges that were involved in this position and the interactions with the providers and colleagues, most of them anyway. I was also taking continuing education courses as rules and regulations were changing fast with the implementation of electronic medical records into the medical field.

During the summer months of 2011 my father started complaining of a "corn flake" being stuck in his throat. "Really Dad, I am pretty sure that a corn flake would dissolve at some point." Hillary and I had both repeatedly told him we thought he needed to go see a doctor. Repeatedly, he would start with the "I don't need to go see a doctor!" After discussion, and then verbalizing these topics to Dad, Hillary and I sat him down and told him that we were not going to argue with him anymore about seeing a doctor. If this is how he wanted to go about life, we were no longer going to take time out of our schedules to sit and waste not only our time, but a doctor's time. Now mind you, he was suffering from early onset vascular dementia brought on by his heart attack, a minor stroke, and prior vascular issues, along with a lifetime of smoking. Despite my siblings' opinions, which were "he knows who we are," they only called maybe once a month to talk about the weather with him. They had no clue what Hillary and I were dealing with on a daily basis. It was a daily problem of inconsideration or stupidity, take your pick. One night in early

August he seemed horse and scratchy, weak, and having that grayish color to him. His smoking had slowed considerably, which he would never give up regardless of what his health status was. Hillary and I agreed we would meet him at the house for dinner and have another little talk. When we arrived at his apartment, we told him that we really thought he should go to the hospital and see what was going on. To our shock and amazement he grabbed his jacket with no complaints of resistance and said okay. We looked at each other in total amazement and with some major concern as this was an unheard-of response.

After several hours, a few scans, and lab work the doctor returned to speak with the three of us. He had a not so positive look on his face and proceeded with "I'm sorry Mr. Dunnigan." That is never a good way to start a conversation. They discovered the "corn flake" was, in fact, an esophageal tumor and it was in an advanced stage. He explained the process in which this would probably go and Dad's response was "I don't want to do anything about it." For the first time in my life I think he made the appropriate choice based on information given. We were told it would be a long and painful process and there was little they could do other than to keep him comfortable. We were given contact information for hospice and released home that evening. This was a heavy night. Hillary decided she was going to stay with him that night and go to classes from there the next morning. He was trying hard to play the tough guy card, but neither one of us was buying it.

The next morning, I went to work and made the hospice appointment. We were scheduled to meet with them at 2 P.M. that same afternoon. I called and let Hillary know, and to "tell Grampa to be ready," I will leave the office early. Hillary apparently went to her morning class and was to meet me at Dad's apartment afterward. Mid-morning, I got an emergency phone call from Hillary. "Mom ... I need you to stay calm, but Grampa is on his way to the hospital, I found him down." She seemed incredibly calm at the time, but at the same time about to lose her shit. I logged out of my computer and flew out of the office stating only I didn't know when I would be back. The girls in the office knew all too well how caring for my father after my mother's passing was weighing heavy on both Hillary and myself in his demands, stubbornness, and lack of insight into how things affected anyone but himself. We both had fulltime jobs and were going to school as well. I believe, in hindsight, that this is a genetic factor, if not a predominately male one, although I have it too, at times. I met Hillary in the Emergency Department less than 10 minutes after her call.

The local hospital was only 2 blocks from my office and the ambulance ride from the apartment less than 10 minutes. Upon my entering the trauma room I attempted to talk with dad. It wasn't good. He had apparently choked on is breakfast, tried to get to the bathroom and fell and hit his head, hard, on the marble vanity and then off the concrete floor. His speech was heavily distorted and I was having a difficult, if not impossible time trying to understand what he was trying to say. Hillary was all over this, understanding what he was trying to tell us and telling me "You need to go tend to the paperwork, I got this." When I left the room to fill out the paperwork, I assured Dad I had his wallet and he could now relax. He was always freaking out thinking someone was out to rip him off or screw him in some manner, even going as far as to instruct Hillary and I who should and should not be in his bedroom on visitation. In any event, Hillary said I was starting to lose my shit. She was right. I was not in a frame of mind that I expected to be in when Dad's time came knocking. Dad was critical and time was limited. Calls were made to my siblings to let them know of Dad's status and the decision was made to just make him as comfortable as possible. This was, lucky for us, a topic for which we had all discussed prior to my mother's passing and a couple of times since. He lost consciousness within a couple of hours after arriving in the ER. After a couple of more hours they moved him up to a room with prognosis of not making it through the night. Hillary and I spent the next 17 hours by his bedside talking to him, holding his hands, waiting for the inevitable. He crossed over at 5 AM the following morning, August 18, 2011.

I wish I could say Dad's passing was a complete shock, but I honestly think he knew there was something far more serious going on than a stuck corn flake. When I would ask him about helping me prepare for Hillary's graduation party coming up in December he would often reply with "if I am still around," like December was years away instead of just a couple of months. The following couple of weeks was a fucking nightmare, and became the disintegration of any relationship I would have with my siblings. We had to empty Dad's apartment of 60+ years of belongings that had been acquired by my parents. It was the goal to leave Dad in familiar surroundings as long as possible and we did, but it came at a very high cost. Everything that couldn't be immediately thrown away or donated to charity, or wasn't already distributed to my siblings at the request of my parents, landed in our home. My living room was floor to ceiling with boxes that would all have to be gone through and separated, dispersed accordingly, or discarded. A project for which was not on the immediate agenda. Would there be a reprieve anytime soon? I was exhausted physically, emotionally, and spiritually.

My parents currently reside on a shelf in the closet of my bedroom. After the behaviors exhibited on the final descent by my siblings, I was not spending another dime to take them back to Maynard for burial. My mother was spot on in her description of what and how my brothers would respond in the event she went first. All I will say here is people should not make death-bed promises they can't possibly, or have no intention of keeping. I am fully aware of the fact that everybody grieves in a different manner. There is a huge difference in grieving and being a complete asshole. Regardless of how your childhood may have played out, this is something to ponder. We all do the best we can with the hands for which we are dealt in life. I was not the biggest fan of the methods in which my father dealt with life, but as I had a child, and my brothers had children, those kids all seemed to adore my dad. For that, I thought, okay he may not have been the greatest for my childhood, but he did the best he could as he knew it coming from an alcoholic background himself. He was a slightly different person when our kids came along, and sober, which made a difference in the way I saw it. His self-absorbed outlook was perhaps inbred as it seems my brothers also have that mentality, the "Big I, little U" syndrome. That was the end of my family unit as I knew it or had hoped it would be on the passing of our parents. Disappointment is an understatement. I was deeply heartbroken at the behavior which was displayed and the treatment for which they threw at me, and after many months of dwelling on this situation I wrote a letter to them all and placed it in the life lessons file of my psyche as best I could. I clearly did not play into any portion of their lives after the death of our parents. It was drilled into my brain that it was not my issue, it was theirs, and therefore, in my best interest to remove the toxicity from my day-to-day life.

The Hits Keep Coming

IN OCTOBER 2011, 6-7 weeks after Dad's passing, I had undergone what turned out to be an unnecessary inguinal hernia operation. I was out of work for six weeks recuperating. This really pissed me off given that this was this PA's second missed call regarding my care. When I questioned her on the first mistake, she got all snotty and snipped she knew best, she had the degree. Now her mistake was thinking that after 40 years of living with Type 1 I didn't know even the basics of my care. I think by now everyone knows how I feel about this type of comment. I could put a "DeR" in front of my name too, that does not make me God or infallible. Her first mistake was attempting to prescribe a Type 2 medications in an attempt to lower my A1c. When I adamantly refused, she said she would note in my chart I was "noncompliant." "You go right ahead and do that, but I will NOT take that med!" When I had followed up with my endocrinologist, she nearly had a stroke and completely agreed with me and my stance, and proceeded to write a letter addressing said situation with the PA's overseeing physician. You would have thought that this encounter and the follow-up from someone who specialized in this disease would have knocked her down a notch or two regarding the intelligence of a patient compared to her degree. Not so much! Needless to say, I underwent the surgery only to have the surgeon tell me he fixed a very small inguinal hernia but felt that it was not my problem and it really did not require surgical intervention at the time. He did, however, remove a "really pissed off lymph node". I returned to work six weeks later with my "nut" as I had fondly nicknamed the bulge in my groin, removed and healing underway. Healing on this OR encounter caused a continuing issue of numbness in the area due to how close the incision was to nerves, being told this is a common occurrence when lymph nodes are removed. Let's add another scar to the map. I'm happy to say that I stopped worrying about what my body looked like after the first two or three surgeries in my life.

With each time an individual is placed under general anesthesia the risks they lay out for you increase. As a diabetic, my risk increases considerably. This was an encounter for which I really didn't need that added risk. I have completely lost track of how many times I have been under anesthesia and I now have a hard time coming out of it without complications. This is a fact Hillary and a couple of others who have witnessed me in a recovery room can attest too. These days I much prefer to be placed under conscious sedation if possible.

On December 5th 2011, my friend Deb-Deb and I headed off to Las Vegas where we had tickets to see a nationally known psychic medium. Yes, I do have a belief in this sort of realm and it goes way back to childhood and that woman who hovered on the ceiling with me. My mom and I also shared outlooks and opinions of the realm of the afterlife, metaphysical readings, along with the spirituality of various cultures. Deb and I had a blast as cheap dates. It was exciting, and with all the losses we had shared together over the past couple of years we felt for sure that "someone would come through and make a little noise." Well, not one spirit showed up for us, but the entire audience received a copy of his latest book and we got our photo taken with him at a meet and greet. In hindsight, you would think if he was really good he would have sensed some impending doom. I'm just saying, as in the next week upon returning to work, my life would change again in a split second, forever, in ways I could never have imagined.

The Hit that Changed My World

UPON MY RETURN to work after the hernia surgery, I had an appointment with HR to update my benefits and tend to some paperwork regarding my being out on bereavement and sick leave. It's always something. Upon leaving the office the weather was changing, it was after all mid-December. It was currently raining. As I was making my way home along Highway 89, the rain changed to a sleety snow mixture. Traffic had come to a crawl as I was about to enter Chino Valley town limits when I saw this car coming at me at a high rate of speed and somewhat erratically. I contemplated trying to speed up to try and avoid what I saw coming but there was no place for me to go with traffic already slow and stopped in the direction for which I was traveling. It would have been an incredible risk. As traffic began to move, all of a sudden everything went into slow motion as I saw this vehicle coming at me spinning! BOOM, lights out!!!

Honestly, I don't recall the moment of impact, only the sound, but I relive that sound and sensation of the hit on a regular basis. I don't know if I passed out, blacked out, or what they call it, but when I opened my eyes, all I saw was a form of thick, white smoke. It turned out to be whatever is given off when an airbag deploys. My leg was throbbing, my hands hurt, I no longer had my glasses on and I was a bit dazed, unsure of what had just transpired. My first response was to get my ass out of the car. I am not a fan of fire and I thought my ass was on fire and the last place I wanted to be was in that car. I didn't even realize when throwing my weight about the door that I was now off the road and in the ditch. I stood on the side of the road shaking and all I saw was chaos and commotion. I am not even really sure how long it took for anyone to realize I had been in that dark blue sedan. I was eventually tended to by EMTs and taken to the hospital via ambulance. I do recall being totally petrified, completely frozen at the thought of being placed into the ambulance, as the last place I wanted to be was in a moving vehicle during these winter conditions. In the ambulance they had cut off my Harley Davidson Denim and cut up the seams of my jeans. I recall telling one of the techs "you better not cut those boots!" This would become a humor release, but not for many, many months afterward.

The rest is sort of a blur. The ER encounter was more than a blur, but fortunately Hillary was in the ER with the neighbor having drove her to the scene of the accident, and then onto the hospital. With that being said, I am going to allow Hillary to give her take on the accident along with the months that follow. Again, life as I knew it, or as I had hoped it may have gone in regard to my up and coming career change as a medical coder, was over. Dead … and I wished on many occasions in the months to come, that I was too.

Accident Aftermath

I GUESS I was home a couple of weeks with what ER defined as contusions. I had been seen by my PCP and an orthopedic guy, and sent back to the ER within a week of the hit. When it came time to go back to work I was a mental case. How was I supposed to get to work? How was I supposed to do my job? I tried, day after day as I was okayed to go back to work four hours per day for the first month. It really wasn't working out well. By the time I got to work after the 30-minute drive I was overly anxious, panicked. With all that anxiety came excruciating headaches. Crushing headaches that matched the body pain and my vision was so fucked up it was difficult to maintain my balance, never mind try and read notes and use my computer screens. I had been to see my ophthalmologist and he said "mild concussion, it'll pass". I don't think he was really putting forth much effort in this diagnosis. "How many fingers do you see?" Whatever, he didn't listen to me. This would really become a major issue. My job required I do a lot of reading and computer work and multiple numerical codes. I was working with dual screens at the time and it was next to impossible for me to do my job if I could not see to accomplish this. Not only was I having difficulty seeing anything of detail, I couldn't seem to retain fucking anything for more than a nanosecond. Like in the time it took me to read something, it was gone. Like it never even stuck to the board (information) and the constant interruptions by an office mate asking questions was unbearably frustrating. I was growing increasingly more irritated and frustrated, outright angry.

I was becoming more and more livid at the entire situation and with that came depression. Where was I? Who was I? What the fuck was I still doing here? This can't be my life …? In the first three months post-accident I had seen and was under the care of numerous doctors as well as six weeks of physical therapy. My neurologist stated that if after three months I had not made progress than that was probably the "best it was going to get." I kept thinking, "oh, hell no!" I felt like nothing more than a shell of the person I was prior to the accident. An accident for which I was NOT at fault!

I began seeing a therapist who worked with brain injury patients to address the changes, physically and emotionally. The PTSD, the panic, the anxiety, the depression, the vision issues, and the effects all this brain shit was having on my diabetic control. I had lost any control I had obtained after my first stem cell treatment only ten months prior.

I have been incredibly blessed with the individuals who have come into my life since my accident and the genuine caring they put forth in looking out for my best interests. Sally, my therapist, whom I saw once a week in the beginning was picking up on the vision issues and referred me to an eye doctor who specialized in TBIs. He worked with a lot of veterans who were returning from service with TBIs and/ or PTSD, which they also diagnosed , again, after the accident. After this consult with Dr. G, I was to embark on 18 grueling months of vision therapy. I had never even heard of vision therapy, but I am happy to say I can't imagine where I would be today if I hadn't had access to this therapy. The guidance, support, and encouragement "don't give up, you're doing an amazing job" or worse, "I don't think I could cope with all you are dealing with," was being drilled into me by these wonderful professionals who took great pride and passion in what they do, and those like me, who must endure to survive. I am by no means special when it comes to those fighting to survive and maintain a semblance of life.

It was about this time I really started to realize what an impact I took to my brain and the effect it was taking on my blood sugar control that I had achieved from my first adipose stem cell treatment. The brain controls every response in one's body, and I was no exception. Vision therapy was once a week, for 30 minutes, and we began to see a direct correlation between using and conditioning my brain to see straight and drops in my blood sugars. Within 30 minutes of leaving therapy I would not only have a headache that felt like someone was driving an ice pick through the center of my head, but I would become incredibly thirsty and my blood sugar would crash. It was a wasted day by any stretch of the imagination, as I would basically wind up asleep for the rest of the day. I slept a LOT!

Now, we were originally told that improvement would show its face within three months of injury. I had hit the three month mark only to find myself still confused, unfocused, always with a headache, and unable to maintain any sort of fluid conversation. I had no sense of humor as I couldn't follow the simplest of conversations. I also had little to no blood sugar control. That fact in itself really pissed me off, and I was angry given how much progress I had made after the stem cell treatment. About this time, two-three months out, I was relieved of my job duties not being able to function at the capacity needed to keep up and without the mistakes that could cost the organization. I was no longer an asset, but a liability.

Far too many people had been witness to the positive changes in my health and appearance since my first stem cell treatment and had been discussing how another round of treatment may help with my brain function. Again, we were told any healing would take place in the first three months. About this time a very generous donor came forward to fund a second stem cell treatment. I was humbled beyond comprehension. Why? I still have a hard time believing that my existence makes that much of an impact on others, especially to strangers and friends, but not my family. It has been explained to me that my drive, determination, perhaps stupidity in the face of adversity encourages others not to give up on life. I am inspiring! Hillary and I made the trip, this time to California, for another round of stem cell treatment. It was already March 2012 and I had no recollection of where the time had gone, or what had taken place in that time since December 13, 2011. In a nanosecond I could be lost regardless of current situation.

On the following pages you will read of Hillary's recollection of the happenings post-accident and how it affected her life. It was a very emotional time for both of us, as well as those who were close to us and followed closely with love, support, and a sense of helplessness at times. This upheaval after all the losses had a really powerful impact on a lot of lives. It is often said that when people feel helpless that they retreat. I understand that all too well now. I continue to stay pretty secluded to this day. I am just not comfortable in crowds or public places as I was once upon a time.

Hillary's Outlook on the Situation

ON DECEMBER 11, 2011, I was supposed to start the next stage of my life as a college graduate. I was graduating from college with my Associates of Applied Nursing, and I was excited to finally have reached graduation! I had worked so hard, literally day and night, working not only as a full-time nursing student during the day, but working as a CNA at the local hospital on the night shift for the past three years to get through school. My mom was so proud; she had planned a big party to follow our ceremony with a big group of our friends to celebrate. It seemed like she had been cooking, cleaning, and doing yard work for days! Of course when the party actually came she was stressed but seemed to enjoy herself, while also enjoying all of the company who had come out to wish me well in my new career. I distinctly remember her telling myself and a group of my friends at about 9:30 that night that it was time to put out the fire in the pit out back and "wrap it up or take it somewhere else before the neighbors call the cops." In her defense, she wasn't trying to be a kill joy, we were a bit more than a few beers in, and getting a bit loud.

What I didn't know when I graduated was that I was about to go from being a full-time nursing student to a full-time live in nurse. Two days after my graduation, on December 13, while I was sitting on our couch in the living room watching a movie at about 4:30 in the afternoon I got a call from my mom. When I answered, her voice was hysterical and I knew something was very wrong. "Hillary, I just wrecked the fucking car! I don't want you to leave the house! I'm okay! My leg hurts so bad!" I went into full blown panic! What the fuck was she talking about don't leave the house? As I tried to keep my cool, I asked her, "What do you mean you wrecked the car? Are the police there? Are you sure you're okay? My mind was racing. As I simultaneously hung up the phone and pulled on my boots, I was praying as hard as my soul would allow that my mom really was alright. I had already lost six people in my life since my senior year in high school, and I was not ready to lose the one person in the world that I was closest to. I ran as fast as my legs, which felt like JELLO by the way, would take me, across the street to our neighbor's house and started frantically pounding on their front door. When they answered, I didn't even say hello. I just blurted out, "Mom was in an accident, she said the car is totaled and not to leave the house, I need a ride to the hospital!" No questions asked, he said, "Gimme a sec, and go get a jacket." I had run across the street in the snow in a t-shirt, but I hadn't even noticed. When I came back out of the house, our neighbor was waiting for me next to their car ready to go. By the time we got to the intersection just before where my mom had told me she had "wrecked the car" the police were shutting down the highway. Shutting down the highway is never a good sign when there is an accident, and my mom was down there! I was told to stay in the car as we pulled off the road. Mike got out and said he was going to see what he could find out. I watched as he walked across the street to talk to the officer that was directing traffic, it didn't look like he was getting anywhere. I opened the car door and stood up, hoping that if the officer knew I was a family member they would have to let us through. We were not so lucky. We were forced to get back in the car, and take the long way around town to the hospital, and the entire ride I prayed. At one point the only thing that could distract me from the horrible thoughts that had been racing through my head since hanging up the phone with my mom was a pair of boots; a pair of Justin cowboy boots that I had bought mom the day before. I had been looking at these boots for her for weeks, because they had a good amount of tread on the sole so she wouldn't slip on the ice, but I knew she would be able to wear thick socks to keep her feet warm in the snow. I had spent almost half of my graduation money on these new boots for her, and she had told me that her leg hurt. All I kept thinking as a distraction was, those paramedics better not cut those brand new $160 boots off of her fucking foot! The insane thought that I was worried about a pair of boots made me start laughing, and in turn, Mike looked at me like I was nuts. When I explained, he started laughing too.

When we got to the hospital, I explained to the emergency room tech at the triage desk that my mom was in an accident and was being brought in by ambulance. She said that because of the weather, the ambulance wasn't even there yet! We beat the ambulance to the hospital. How does that even happen? So I took a seat in one of the waiting room chairs, something that as a hospital staff member I didn't do well, especially when I am anxious. A few minutes later, the tech called me back up to the desk. She told me that the ambulance wasn't here yet but that she wasn't going into a Critical Care room. A very good sign, so I tried to relax a little bit. A few minutes more passed before I was allowed to go back into the Emergency Department and see my mom. When I got into the room, my mom was conscious, laying on a back board, and had a collar around her neck to keep her from moving her head, nothing out of the ordinary for a motor vehicle accident. I was very relieved to see this, until the doctor walked into her room. She had truly only been in the building maybe ten minutes at the most, the doctor came in and his words shocked me. "She's neurologically stable, get her off the board, lose the C-collar, put an immobilizer on her leg and let her go." I'm sorry? Did you not take trauma 101 in medical school you arrogant asshole? Unless you're Superman with the X-ray vision crap, you cannot prove that she is neurologically stable, and have not followed standard protocol for that type of injury, but I'm no doctor, just a nurse. At the time I was just a new grad nurse, who hadn't yet sat for my state boards, and was in shock over a traumatic family situation. I knew something was wrong with how that doctor dealt with my mom's situation, and I said nothing. I have felt guilty about that for a long time. If I had said something that night about the treatment of my mom, if I had insisted on a CT scan or a spinal series of X-rays before they had released my mom from the hospital, maybe she wouldn't have had all the problems that she has as a result. Maybe it wouldn't have made a difference, but a nurse is supposed to be a patient advocate, and right then I didn't advocate for my mom. I let that doctor discharge her from the ER, we managed to squish her into the back seat of a Ford Mustang, and Mike took us home. Again, what I didn't know was that just two days later I was going to have to pull up my big girl pants and start advocating for my mom.

Two days after the accident my mom and I were both lying on the couch, her knee looked hideous, and it was so swollen that the immobilizer was painful to wear. She had a mass the size of a softball where her knee should have been, and it was a horrible shade of purple from bleeding under the skin. As she stood up from the couch and hobbled into the kitchen, I heard her stop. She didn't say anything, and I couldn't hear her doing anything, so I got up. As I walked into the kitchen, she looked at me puzzled. I asked her, "are you okay?" and she just continued to look at me. When she finally responded, it was a red flag in the nursing portion of my mind, "What did I get up for again?" How was I supposed to know what she got up for? She hadn't said anything, she just got up and gimped her way in here, then she didn't even answer the question, she asked one. I told her to get dressed because I was taking her back to the doctor. When we got to her primary care doctor about 30 minutes later without an appointment, I told the receptionist at the desk about the accident and how her mental state had changed since then, and we were put on the list to see the doctor. Her normal doctor wasn't there that day, but her partner was, and lucky for us I had worked with him before at the hospital and he knew that I knew what I was talking about. The doctor told me that I needed to take her back to the ER for a CT scan and

X-rays, and that he would be calling ahead to let them know that we were on our way. Now my mom is not a fan of the hospital, rightfully so. So, when she has no objection to a visit to the Emergency room, another red flag goes up, and this time she went without a word of dispute. When we got to the hospital, we told the staff at the triage desk that we had been sent from the doctor's office and that he was supposed to have called ahead. She notified the nurse and we only sat in the waiting room for a few minutes. When we got into a room and the doctor came in, I had a hard time keeping my composure. I had had time to calm down from the accident, and I was in full blown advocacy mode at this point. Although this was not the same doctor that had treated mom so poorly on the night of the accident, I was not about to let another doctor do the same. I insisted on a full neurological exam to accompany the CT scan and X-rays. When we got all the test results back the doctor came back in, she had a closed traumatic head injury, a concussion. The doctor provided all the crappy patient education paperwork that the hospital is required to provide at discharge, told us if her mental state changed drastically to bring her back, but that it could take up to a year for her to come back to her normal mental state. They sent us home again.

Over the next few months, I learned just how serious a concussion can become. In school, they teach us that traumatic brain injuries can alter a person's personality, but something you truly just can't fully understand until it happens to you. My mom became increasingly short-tempered, constantly tired, angry about little things, and forgetful. She didn't understand jokes that she would have normally understood, she yelled at me about little things that would have never bothered her before, and she was angry about things that were at the time out of my control. My mom wasn't my mom anymore. She had become a shell of the person I knew so well, with an empty anger and frustration inside that I could do little to help with. She would sit in the exact same spot on the couch for hours with her laptop on her lap, not saying a word, while I went to work, did the grocery shopping, did laundry and the dishes. When she would get up from the couch, if there were dishes in the sink or laundry still in the dryer, she would start screaming at me, "This is your house too you know!" and "You never do anything at home, you always have something better to do! You want to be treated like an adult; maybe you should start acting like one!" I was acting like one! I had now become the parent. My mom's car accident had inflicted a level of depression on both of us that neither one of us was prepared for. I was supposed to be starting the next chapter of my life, and instead I felt like I had to stay home and take care of my mom. How was I supposed to start my life if I felt so responsible for another person? I wasn't a parent yet, I shouldn't have to be responsible for my parent.

As my mom's mood changes continued, we began fighting on what seemed like a daily basis, about stupid things, like the fact that I didn't buy her any "cupcakes with the squiggles" while I was at the grocery store, or that I washed her laundry but didn't fold it. A comment that would have normally gotten a good laugh out of my mom before the accident now didn't even seem to register in her mind, and things that would have just irritated her before the accident were now making her go ballistic. This wasn't just a car accident that totaled a car and caused some minor injuries. Even though no lives were taken in this accident, it ruined lives!

Over the course of the six months following the accident, I got my first nursing job; it was in the Phoenix area, about two hours away from our home. I would spend the several days I was scheduled to work in Phoenix, and drive home on my days off to check on my mom and make sure that she had everything she needed. My mom became increasingly depressed, whether due to my not being around, the stress of our relationship, or the fact that she could no longer mentally handle doing a lot of the things she was used to doing, I don't know. It seemed like days would go by and she would always be in the same spot on the couch, in the same clothes staring off mindlessly. Along with the not being able to focus on everyday tasks, she was having a very difficult time keeping her blood sugar stable. It didn't matter if she was eating healthy food or total crap, or if she checked her sugar 20 times a day, her blood sugars became out of control again.

After the first stem cell treatment, her blood sugars became so much more stable than they had been in years. She was able to feel the symptoms when her blood sugar was dropping before it became dangerous. After the car accident, and the injury she sustained, her body needed so many extra calories to try and heal, that her blood sugar would drop without warning. Her brain needed extra carbohydrates and protein to heal, and she couldn't seem to eat enough to maintain her stability. We made several trips to the emergency room because of the instability of her blood sugar levels. The seemingly constant mood swings, always worrying about her blood sugars and if she would be able to take care of them, and the increasing tension in our relationship began to weigh heavily on me as a new nurse. I, too, quickly became depressed, avoiding being at home as much as possible. When I was home, we would fight and I would end up storming out of the house or locking myself in my room, not a healthy situation for either one of us to be living in, and certainly not the supportive and therapeutic environment that my mom needed to heal. So a little over a year after my mom's accident, I got a job offer, packed my truck, and moved to Colorado. Problem solved, right? Wrong!

When I moved to Colorado, I didn't know a soul. I had never been there before, had no idea about the neighborhood that I had just rented my first apartment in, nobody to help me move my heavy stuff in, no TV. Hell, I didn't even have a mattress because I had gotten rid of the one I had at my mom's house. In my mind at the time, it was an escape from the responsibility of "taking care of my mom," and an adventure all at the same time. I liked the new job I had. I quickly made some good friends and I started going out and trying new things. I was homesick for a while, and I came home to visit within the first six months of my move. Although I was happy to be out on my own, I was heartbroken that my mom wasn't able to make the trip with me. She couldn't see the look on my face when

I unlocked the door to my first apartment, or help me decorate or have a meal with me, and I know it broke her heart too. I missed being able to yell down the hall to her when something goofy happened, and because I was a broke new grad with irregular work hours, I couldn't afford internet or cable, or any of the luxuries, so we talked on the phone every day. After a while, I began to get depressed again. Whether it was related to being homesick, or only having a few friends who had lives of their own, or my horribly irregular work schedule, or just the fact that I was still worrying about my mom, I can't say. What I do know is that I saw myself start to go down a road that I promised myself as a child of an alcoholic I would never go down. I realized that I had been drinking nearly every night, whether I was out with friends or home alone it didn't matter as long as I didn't have to be up for work early.

About a year after I moved to Colorado, I found out that I was pregnant. When I made that phone call to my mom, I felt like the biggest disappointment of her life. I was so disappointed in myself and I knew she felt the same. I had had an image of how I wanted my life to go in my head since I was young, and my life had not followed that path for what seemed like an eternity. When I found out I was pregnant, that was my wake-up call. That was a higher power of some kind, perhaps my grandmother, slapping me in the face and telling me, "Wake up!! You are the adult now!!" I promised myself that I was going to get my shit together. When I went for my first ultrasound, and I heard my son's little heartbeat in my belly that was all it took. While I know my mom was disappointed in me, she was just as supportive as she would have been at a high school band concert. She flew to Colorado, stayed with me for a month at the end of my pregnancy. She knew how difficult being a single mom was, and being a single mom without a solid support system close by, is even harder. While she offered to let me come home, I refused. I had made the choice to move to Colorado on my own, and I would do what I had to do to support myself and my son. If I failed, I knew she would be there. My son is 8-years old now, I am not a single mother anymore, and I really haven't been since the day he was born because a great guy, a friend of mine from before I was pregnant walked into our lives and blessed us, and my mom loves my son more than I could have ever imagined possible.

I have been in Colorado for 4 years now, and I still worry about my mom every single day. I have learned to not freak out when she doesn't answer the phone all the time, or respond to a text message within a certain period of time, but I do still worry. Shortly after moving, I called her 9 times in a 24-hour period, texted her multiple times, and emailed her, all without a response or acknowledgement that she was still alive. Due to the fact that it is VERY unusual for us to go without communicating for this long, I became more concerned than usual, and I called the police. I asked them to do a welfare check on her stating that she was a diabetic and we speak regularly and I hadn't heard from her in almost two days. Let me just say, I will never be doing that again, unless I have serious reason to believe she is incapacitated. She was fine, and due to the other fact that I worked in a prison at the time, and an officer showed up on her doorstep asking if I was her daughter, she just about had a heart attack. She thought he was showing up to tell her I had been attacked at work or something horrible had happened to me. Oops.

When my mom first asked me to write about our lives after the accident, I was very reluctant. I viewed her as this fragile, moody, shell of my mother for a long time after the wreck. I was afraid to write what I really felt because I thought that somehow, after all we have been through together that I was going to hurt her feelings. Although some of these things may be difficult for her to read, I know now that they are never going to change her opinion of me. I know how much my mom gave up to help shape me into the person that I am today, and I know that I wouldn't be that person without her influence, good or bad, at any given time. I also realize now, that getting her story out, about her lack of quality healthcare, or inability to utilize healthcare that could really be life changing, or what a traumatic brain injury can actually do to a person, their personality, and their family, is more important that worrying about if I hurt her feelings for a little while. I know she will get over it, especially if her story turns out to help and/or support another person or family going through similar circumstances. And, mom if I have hurt your feelings, I am sorry, but you did tell me to "Be brutally honest." So, there you go – brutal honesty.

Healthcare and Justice

I HAVE LITTLE to no memory of how I located an attorney to handle the accident. It was blatantly obvious right out of the gate that the insurance industry was out to screw me and I was in no condition to even attempt to navigate this bumpy terrain. I retained, what I thought at the time, was a competent attorney from a large Phoenix firm. I was to work with the son of one of the founding partners at O&H. This, when all is said and done, would be a very hard lesson learned. In a nutshell: Insurance companies don't give a shit about you and in my opinion, neither do your so-called hired attorneys. My understanding to this day is this ~ If you will be paid a hefty amount of money to look out for my best interest, to do the right thing in getting those responsible for altering my life, to make things right, to compensate me for all my losses, then this gentleman failed on a large scale. All of those people who took this hell ride with me over the first three years post-accident kept telling me "You need a new attorney" "What's this guy doing besides stringing you along?" It was a nightmare! A pure and total living hell on earth.

My sense of time and recollection will never be the same. I can pull tidbits of information, trivia, etc. out of my ass dating back to childhood or 25 years, but ask me what I did last week, yesterday, or even an hour ago and nada, nothing. Useless! This is by far the most frustrating of my adjustments. The constant repetitiveness of life ... you've seen the movie, "Ground Hogs Day"? This was now a large part of my make up and I am sad to say, there were individuals who could not cope with my changes and, therefore, went by the wayside. Sorry, but this could happen to anyone. ANYONE, rich, poor, educated, established, anyone. To have life as you know it taken away from you by an individual who not only was the cause of this change, but is not even held accountable for his actions, is the utmost in disgusting, a true injustice. Many would take on this outlook toward my attorney, and a few others who played a major role in stringing along the process.

The legal case against the insurance company of the other party was dragged out over two years. In this time frame along with loss of my brain function, vision issues, and decline in my health status both physically and emotionally, I also lost my job, my health insurance, and ultimately Hillary and I lost our home which we purchased together in 2007. All the while, wonder boy the attorney is telling me "it would be devasting for you to lose your health insurance." No shit Sherlock! He became driven by a $1-million-dollar umbrella policy, for which he never even made an attempt to chip into. I am still dumbfounded as to where he thought I was getting the money to survive. I was a single, white woman under the age of 65, with no minor children. I did not qualify for ANY state subsidiaries and the application for SSDI could and would take two-plus years as well.

I was, by the grace of God, blessed with some very loving and giving friends, who would tend to my financial needs the entire time this asshole was finding any means possible to drag this out, instead of getting to the bottom of it. Instead of putting up the fight he should have, he wimped out. I had an ill feeling about this guy from the beginning, but was also questioning my own abilities to cope in the real-world situation. I have always had a hard time with anyone who can't make eye contact when speaking with someone else. It's a trust issue for me. Needless to say, I, nor anyone in my circle felt this guy did $80+ thousand dollars worth of work on my behalf, or in my best interest. Word of mouth is a powerful form of advertisement, good or bad, and this establishment is NOT a good place and I will more than happily share that firm name, O&H in full with anyone who inquires, and I have several times already. What I find incredibly ironic is that the accident lawyer was so quick to bad mouth my Social Security attorney. Although somewhat flamboyant and loud, at least my SS lawyer went to bat and fought for me, especially when they were dragging their feet in making my benefits a reality. I do, after all, suffer with a chronic disease for which is not only a juggling act to maintain, it is quite pricey and at this point no longer have the capacity to maintain a viable work status. I truly believe the guy was just waiting on me to die.

After Hillary had moved to Colorado there was not much time left before I would have to vacate the premises of our home which had already fallen into foreclosure. I really had no plan other than waiting on funds to help put my life back on some sort of path. That wouldn't happen for another 6-8 months. With the help of friends, who would later turn out not to be, what was left of my belongings were put into storage. Luckily for me, I had placed what I felt was most valuable to me, in a storage facility that Hillary had prior to her move. There was not a lot left after we sold off most of the big stuff in a yard sale. Again, I felt beyond deflated. An empty shell of a being attempting to see a life that was currently non-existent, no future in sight.

In May 2013, I was homeless. I would spend a couple of weeks with friends in Phoenix, a couple of weeks "house sitting" for a cousin who lived locally, and then the call that eased my mind and spirit. Like a gift from the Gods, I received an email from a former coworker who was currently out of the country and would be until December. He informed me that he had renters in his home, who would vacating six months prior to agreed time. He offered me his home until December. A win-win situation for both us, or so he stated. I had a temporary roof over my head and could keep my dog, Maggie, with me, and he had someone to keep an eye on the property. The receipt of that email brought me to tears and made me weak with humble thanks of friendship. So with all my worldly belongings in my truck I began a six month run at vagabond living.

While in this little hideaway, I would go through paperwork and discard anything that was no longer needed. I continued in my therapies, both vision therapy, cognitive, and psychological therapy. It was a very dark time for me, and there were often moments of just not wanting to go on. I slept a lot! I often wondered why? Why was I still here? Why was I able to get out of that car walking and talking? All the "whys" had to be pushed to the back of my mind as I couldn't give up knowing how very generous and supportive certain people were to my survival and recovery. I was, however, beyond exhausted and frustrated, both physically and emotionally. Those dark times were something I really wanted to touch on in my story, how they play with the diabetes and the hurdles that are produced, but maybe in the second coming. I am hoping that you got the picture of stress related complications in the earlier part of my journey. Some would say that most of my life has been stress filled. That my humor and methods of coping with life's dirty little deeds that many never experience is what make me a tough cookie, a surviving spirit. It still plays a major role in the destruction of a person's well-being and overall health.

I moved into my forever home with few possessions in October 2013. We emptied out the storage unit, and I waited weeks for the return of my belongings from the so-called friends. Much to my disappointment, I didn't get it all back and that "friendship" dissolved quite quickly when confronted and I got nothing but avoidance, no eye contact, or reasonable explanation. I really should listen to people who see things before I do, and accept them as truth. These individuals apparently were only out to see what they could get for free, or close to it, with no real caring of me or my situation. That hurt deeply. I can be a slow learner in the school of human nature.

When my Social Security benefits finally became reality and I was awarded the retroactive monies dating back to the original filing, two years earlier, I was able to not only furnish my little bungalow, but I was able to secure another round of stem cell treatment. Yes, I booked round three to take place in early December 2014. Again, I couldn't have asked for better care and treatment. I was walking the beach within hours of my procedure and feeling great in hopes of further improvements in my health status.

Where I Am Today

IT HAS TAKEN me several years to get this story into a format for which others may find it not only a flowing dialog, but inspiring, informative, and perhaps even a tad entertaining.

It's been a good number of years since my last stem cell treatment. I wish I could find a means to try one more time as my health has seriously deteriorated over the last 4-5 years. I have come to the conclusion that to maintain all the positive effect I get from these treatments I would have to undergo a treatment every couple of years. That is just not feasible on a fixed income. I no longer have the networking ability to fundraise. There are arenas for which people can seek help in these matters of healthcare and treatment options, but so few are openly shared through hospitals, doctors, or government outlets. It is up to those of us who have encountered these types of situations to share information with others. The struggles that families can come upon in the midst of a medical emergency or living with a chronic or terminal disease can be life changing and most devastating. Sadly, many people die before they get the help they need. Not only that dark end, there is the money involved, being sucked to the brink of bankruptcy just to undergo treatments and maintain monthly medical costs.

In September 2016, I went to Washington, DC to testify before the FDA/NIH on the regulations of stem cell treatments. It was an exciting time for me having recently spent 5-days in the hospital with a blood clot in my intestine for which caused an acute bout of ischemic colitis. That incident right there could have killed me. Flying was a fear for me, but I had worked so long and hard on my speech and spoke so passionately about the use of stem cells for many diseases since my first infusion in 2010 in Mexico that I had to pull up my big girl panties. I am a huge fan, and a firm believer of bringing these treatments to use in the United States with less restriction. How much positive outcome and response do they need to justify the use of stem cell treatments as a normal route of therapy for so many? My answer to this question is this: Why would any pharmaceutical company, the FDA and other agencies want to cure a disease, disorder, syndrome, etc.,? We, the patients, are nothing more than cash cows for big pharma. The results are out there. As I have stated many times prior, the political stronghold over our healthcare must stop! Pharmaceuticals are getting rushed through and approved, and treatments involving the use of stem cells are being held back to see who can get their hands in on it, and who will make the most money from it. All this red tape while many people are dying waiting on the promises of the powers that be. I've been waiting 50 years!! Fifty years of waiting, and listening, and reading of a potential cure for Type 1. Every single ray of hope usually shot down with a comment like "it's still 10 years out" or "it will begin clinic trial in X number of years," and the clinical trial process can take a LOT of years. Talk about stringing along the public. There are many, many passionate scientists, researchers, doctors, and staffs who are working diligently to make progress all the while the FDA is throwing up roadblocks at every intersection. I do agree that there is fraud in the stem cell arena, as in any arena, there are unscrupulous individuals who do not have the patients' best interest at heart. My advice – DO YOUR RESEARCH!

I still struggle with short-term memory problems, I tire easily, I often sleep for what seems like days, and yet have sleep issues at times when I can't sleep at all. If I exert myself physically for one day, I usually pay for 3-5 days in the physical exhaustion and pain department, which brings a sense of empty brain fog and sense of disorientation.

I have muscle issues where my legs feel weak and wobbly. My vision has its ups and downs with the exacerbation of diabetic retinopathy and having cataracts removed, which are part of a diabetic laundry list of complications. I still suffer with body pain from the accident, for which this will not doubt continue to progress as I age. As if living with neuropathy, fibromyalgia and sequelae of the accident, I have lost two inches in height due to my spine deteriorating, bone on bone in many areas, which is painful, and take no pain medication for a number reasons, the stem cell treatments did amazing things for my pain levels. I am surviving but believe there is much room for improvement, however, my expectations have been lowered with all the bullshit in which must be shoveled to get what one needs most. Added to all the red tape, comes out-of-pocket expenses for such supplements, medications, and insulin pump/CGM supplies. That doesn't leave a lot of extra funds, if any, to enjoy something like a vacation once in a while.

My Opinions and Hopes for the Future

MUCH TO THE disappointment of some, I don't feel as though my time here on earth is destined to go on for a lot of years ahead. To those I say this. I did my best. I fought as long as I could with what I had. My body saddled with a brain injury for which I have never quite felt as I did prior to my accident, along with the years of Type 1 and a myriad of other afflictions now, I did okay given the journey. Would I have changed any of it? Maybe early on … but, if I had not survived the early years of dysfunction, or the long abusive relationship, I would not be the woman I am today or have the most amazing, beautiful daughter anyone could ask for. I do believe that things happen for a reason and that those happening are meant to teach us. I've learned that there are some people and situations that are just best to walk away from because there are many people in this world who don't give a shit about anyone but themselves and will use any means to obtain that goal. I've learned that there are people that regardless of how much they have, are never happy. They get off on complaining / bitching, blaming others for anything that may be lacking in their own lives. Those that will take credit for things that they never played a role in, only to make themselves look good. To those I say karma will get you in the end. For myself, I never claimed to be perfect. I am human, and for the most part, I have always played by those rules of "treat others as you would want to be treated". If you don't like me, stay the fuck away from me. It's that simple. I've been described as harsh, brass, and rude. I see it as this: I say what most people are thinking, so if that makes me the bad, oh, well, I can live with that. I have never been one who practices "political correctness". I had a brother-in-law who would often laugh and comment, "You're such a nonconformist". I will die fighting for what I believe in, and if you happen to be an individual who did me or a loved one wrong, or you practice ill or unethical behaviors, you will eventually feel the burn of your actions with no help from me. I will continue to advocate for the use of stem cell treatments and therapies for those Americans who can benefit. With the passing of the 21st Century Cures Act, I have great faith that this may become a reality for which I will live to see and perhaps participate in. That is my prayer, my continued hope. Even with prayers and continued hope though, I will eventually die, as we all will, but my body is tired and with so many years of broken promises in the field of medicine, and the status of our healthcare today, hope can only last so long.

My methods of coping with life as it was handed to me, comes down to the simple practice of doing what is right, not intentionally going out of the way to inflict pain or suffering. I sleep very well at night regarding my inner self and my conscience being clear. I have no doubt that I have inflicted an amount of pain on certain people as a means of protecting myself, and later my daughter, but, if you can't take it, you shouldn't be dishing it out in the first place. I have spent long periods of time speaking to the "Big Guy" as to help in guidance, strength, or when it may be okay for me to call it quits. In all reality, there will come a time that my life just ends. I hope and pray that it is a quick passing. I have often felt like the cat, and I have already played out my nine lives, having dodged many bullets. That comment that I heard as a 9-year-old girl of "she'll never see 21" has played itself over and over in my lifetime and here I am 38 years after that fact and I am still blessed with a fairly independent existence.

For that I am truly blessed and forever grateful!

Along with the sense of spirituality, comes my dark sense of humor. I do find a means of laughing even in the darkest of situations. I've been applauded and reprimanded for this action of laughter. By the medical community, from the time I was a child, a teenager, a young woman, and as an adult, been told my humor has served me well in that it allows for a much needed stress release. Only certain people, actually get this about me. To medical staff for whom I have made their jobs challenging, i.e., inability to get in an IV line, holding up the OR ~ I am grateful for your feeding my dark, sometimes vulgar scenarios. In my opinion, most medical staff have this same warped outlook, so when they can laugh with me, it makes the whole ordeal, whatever that may be, a little easier to cope with. I have been told by many that have witnessed some of my medical escapades, that my ability to laugh has inspired them to be stronger. Inspiration is a term I find hard to apply where my own journey is concerned. I am trying to live my life as best I can with the working pieces for which I have been given. There are far more people in this world who suffer with disease, whatever it may be, and make my struggles small in comparison. However, with that being said, it warms my heart to know that I have the ability to make others look to something bigger and better. To say it is okay to plow forward in search of a better life, better treatments, to be a voice for those who can't seem to speak for themselves. I am, if nothing else determined to advocate for stem cell treatments as a means of treatment until cures can be found. It only makes sense to me.

Stem cell treatments have been a life saving alternative for me. Far better than the numerous pharmaceuticals for which I've been placed on over the years. With all those drugs comes side effects, mix a bunch of them together and you are asking for trouble on so many levels people just don't comprehend those dangers. Doctors don't seem to communicate (my opinion and experience) , and often are trained to give a line of defense in regard to new treatments and alternative options. We, as patients, or advocates of loved ones, must be forthcoming in our concerns. Doctors are not Gods! Medicine is science. Praying for miracles comes in many disguises.

I have been fortunate to have encountered more decent, passionate doctors and researchers for whom appreciate my outlook and are willing to share their knowledge. I remain hopeful that I will live long enough to not only receive another stem cell treatment, but to see the future come alive in giving people of the United States a better quality of life and stop raping the American public in high hospital bills, treatments that will not work for everyone, and the high cost of medications to treat such diseases. These occurrences I have witnessed first hand with my parents care as well as my own.

I hope that the story of my journey, in its condensed form as I spared a LOT of dirty details, has helped to open an avenue for which you were unaware, or just curious about. If you are interested in stem cell treatments, do your research. There are many areas for which clinical trials are already in place. There are other countries that are in many aspects far ahead of the United States in using stem cells as a means of treatment and regenerative medicine. They have been practicing these methods for decades. Investigate! Do not become the desperate individual who will be taken advantage of. Just like we don't all respond the same to any given medication, we can't all expect to respond the same to stem cell treatments. Advocate for your own care. There are several states for which the "Right to Try" is law.

My goals include the hope of selling my story to obtain another stem cell treatment and help with outstanding medical debt. To continue to advocate not only for my own health, but for others who may be interested in more advanced means of treatment for so many afflictions that present themselves in today's world.

May you never feel alone in your quest for a better quality of life!